INTELLIGENCE AND COUNTERINTELLIGENCE STUDIES

CURING ANALYTIC PATHOLOGIES

PATHWAYS TO IMPROVED INTELLIGENCE ANALYSIS

INTELLIGENCE AND COUNTERINTELLIGENCE STUDIES

Additional books in this series can be found on Nova's website under the Series tab.

Additional e-books in this series can be found on Nova's website under the e-book tab.

INTELLIGENCE AND COUNTERINTELLIGENCE STUDIES

CURING ANALYTIC PATHOLOGIES

PATHWAYS TO IMPROVED INTELLIGENCE ANALYSIS

OLIVIER C. FITCH
AND
RYAN A. SADLER

NOVINKA
New York

For permission to use material from this book please contact us:
Telephone 631-231-7269; Fax 631-231-8175
Web Site: http://www.novapublishers.com

Additional color graphics may be available in the e-book version of this book.

Library of Congress Cataloging-in-Publication Data

ISBN: 978-1-62618-279-0

Published by Nova Science Publishers, Inc. † New York

CONTENTS

Foreword

Dear reader, my task in this foreword is to shackle your attention to the challenge of getting through Jeffrey Cooper's monograph that follows.

Your attention is deserved because the subject—what we label with deceptive simplicity "intelligence analysis"—is so important and so interesting. The scope of this monograph, like that of the analytic profession, is broad and deep, from support to military operations to divining the inherently unknowable future of mysterious phenomena, like the political prospects of important countries. Jeff Cooper's study, as befits the work of one who has long been an acute observer of the Intelligence Community and its work, is packed with critiques, observations, and judgments. It would be even more satisfying if the study could be further illuminated by clinical case studies of failures and successes. In principle, this lack could be remedied if the hurdle of classification could be cleared. In practice, it cannot currently be fixed because an adequate body of clinical, diagnostic case studies of both successes and failures and lessons learned, particularly from the most relevant, post-Cold War intelligence experience, simply does not now exist. Not surprisingly, Mr. Cooper, along with many other critics and reformers, such as the Silberman-Robb Commission (of which he was a staff member), recommends the institutionalization of a lessons-learned process in our national intelligence establishment. This is but one of a rich menu of admonitions to be found in this study.

Mr. Cooper has provided a good, thematic summary of the main points of his monograph. I shall not attempt to summarize them further in this foreword. But some overview comments are in order.

This study is fundamentally about what I would call the intellectual professionalization of intelligence analysis. It is about standards and practices and habits of mind. It is about inductive (evidence-based) analytical reasoning balanced against deductive (hypothesis-based and evidence tested) reasoning. It extols the value of truly scientific modes of thinking, including respect for the role of imagination and intuition, while warning against the pitfalls of "scientism," a false pretense to scientific standards or a scientific pose without a scientific performance. It talks about peer review and challenging assumptions and the need to build these therapeutic virtues into the analytical process.

Mr. Cooper makes reference to the standards and practices of other professions with a high order of cerebral content, such as law and medicine. Other recognized authors, such as Stephen Marrin and Rob Johnston, have written persuasively on this theme. I am struck by how frequently Mr. Cooper—and others—refers to the example of medicine, especially internal medicine, which has much to offer our discipline. But I am not surprised. When I was very young in this business, I was fretting about its difficulties in the company of my uncle, an old and seasoned physician. He walked to his vast library and pulled out for me a volume, *Clinical Judgment*, by Alvan Feinstein, a work now often cited by intelligence reformers. I later asked my mother, my uncle's younger sister, what made Uncle Walt such a great doctor. Her answer: He always asks his patients at the beginning, "how do you feel?" and he never makes it home for dinner on time. The model of internal medicine is a great one for critical emulation by intelligence analysis: science, training, internship, expertise, experience, and then seasoned judgment, intuition, unstinting diligence, and valued second opinions.

Most of what Mr. Cooper writes about concerns the intellectual internals of good intelligence analysis, i.e., standards, methods, the tool box of techniques, and the vital element of attitude toward understanding and knowledge building. With somewhat less emphasis but to good effect, he also addresses what might be called the environmental internals of the same: training, mentoring, incentives, management, and leadership. It is in this dimension that we must overcome the plague recognized by all informed critics, the tyranny of current intelligence, and restore the value of and resources for deep analysis.

This leads to a consideration of the "externals" of good intelligence analysis. To wit:

The full scope of analysis: This has to be appreciated for things to come out right. Analysis is not just what a hard-pressed analyst does at his desk. It is the whole process of cerebration about the mission and its product. This applies to not only the best answer to a current intelligence question on the table, but to establishing priorities, guiding collection, and, especially, to judging whether the best effort on the question of the day is good enough to support the weight of the situation and the policy decisions that have to be made.

Money and people: There is no gainsaying that a lot of our failings after the Cold War are the fault of resource and personnel cuts while old and new and more equally competing priorities were proliferating. We've got to fortify the bench strength of intelligence analysis. The president has called for that. Without improved practices, however, new resources will be wasted. We press for improved practices; but they need more resources to be implemented effectively.

External knowledge environments: Half a century ago, when the United States came to appreciate that it faced an enigmatic and dangerous challenge from the Soviet Union, it invested seriously in the building of knowledge environments on that subject, in the government, in think tanks, in academia, and in other venues. These external sources of expertise, corrective judgment, and early warning proved vital in keeping us on track with respect to the Soviet problem. We have yet to get serious about building such knowledge environments for the challenges of proliferation and, especially, concerning the great struggle within the world of Islam, from which the main threat of terrorism emerges. Related to this, Mr. Cooper's study properly places great importance on our improving exploitation of open sources.

Information security regimes: We are talking here about a complicated domain from classification to recruitment and clearance systems. What we have is hostile to the task of developing a comprehensive, communitywide knowledge base and operational efficacy in the age of information and globalization. We need to be more open on a lot of things, especially where the original reason for secrecy perishes quickly and the value of openness is great (as during the Cold War in regard to Soviet strategic forces), and to tighten up on secrecy where it is vital, for example, in protecting true and valuable cover.

One final—and perhaps most important—point: Mr. Cooper's study of intelligence analysis is shot through with a judgment that is shared by almost every serious professional I've heard from in recent years. And it applies to collection and other aspects of national intelligence as well. We cannot just rely on the new Director of National Intelligence (DNI) superstructure to put things right with our national intelligence effort. The problems and pathologies that inhibit our performance and the opportunities for radically improving that performance are to be found down in the bowels and plumbing of this largely dutiful ship we call the Intelligence Community, and that is where we must studiously, and with determination, concentrate our efforts and our money.

— Fritz Ermarth[1]

End Note

[1] Fritz Ermarth is a former chairman of the National Intelligence Council; he is now a security policy consultant.

PREFACE

A wide range of problems have contributed to the unease currently pervading the Intelligence Community. A significant number of the most serious problems result from shortcomings in intelligence analysis rather than from defects in collection, organization, or management. The obvious and very public failures exemplified by the surprise attacks of September 11, 2001 and by the flawed National Intelligence Estimate (NIE) of 2002 on Iraqi weapons of mass destruction (WMD) have resulted in a series of investigations and reports that have attempted to identify the causes of those failures and to recommend corrective actions. This book examines and explores the pathways for improved intelligence analysis and curing analytic pathologies in intelligence gathering.

ACKNOWLEDGMENTS

The journey that produced this study owes much to many people. Some of them can be named, others cannot; but all of them have my deepest appreciation and deserve to be acknowledged for their support in this effort. And to my wife Lisa, who can be named— special thanks for putting up with me throughout.

I began to appreciate the depth of the Intelligence Community's analytic problems during a series of research and analysis efforts for various of its components starting in the mid-1990s, and I would like to thank the sponsors of those many efforts even though they cannot be named. Frank Jenkins, General Manager of Science Applications International Corporation (SAIC) Strategies Group, deserves special praise for allowing Fritz Ermarth and me to follow our instincts and start to investigate these issues before the failures became so very public. Particular thanks are owed to Henry Abarbanel for a discussion of the contrasts between the practice of science and that of intelligence analysis, a conversation that prompted me to focus on the deep cultural and process factors that affect analytic efforts rather than on the superficial symptoms and manifestations of the failures.

I owe a debt to Mike May, Dean Wilkening, and Scott Sagan of Stanford University's Center for International Security and Cooperation (CISAC) for inviting me to give a seminar on intelligence issues that forced me to organize and sharpen my concerns into the original briefing on "Analytic Pathologies," and I am truly grateful to both Aris Pappas and Stan Feder for reviewing that lengthy presentation slide by slide. Paul Johnson, Director of the Center for the Study of Intelligence, has my appreciation for an invitation to CSI's 2003 conference on "Intelligence for a New Era in American Foreign Policy"; as do the many intelligence professionals at that conference who helped by bringing their concerns into the open. I want to thank the members of the Marriott Group on the Revolution in Intelligence Affairs, as well as David Kay, Mike Swetnam, Gordon Oehler, and Dennis McBride of the Potomac Institute for providing forums for discussion and for helping me think through these issues with their insider perspectives. Thanks are also owed to several former senior intelligence officials who then pushed me to go beyond diagnosis and address the harder questions of fixing the problems.

I want to thank the Commissioners and my fellow staff members of the President's Commission on the Intelligence Capabilities of the United States Regarding Weapons of Mass Destruction (the Silberman-Robb Commission) for the lengthy opportunity to delve into these issues, examine them in great depth, and analyze them within a truly professional search for understanding. I am also grateful to both the former and the current Program Managers, Lucy Nowell and Rita Bush, of Advanced Research and Development Activity's (ARDA's) Novel Intelligence from Massive Data (NIMD) Program, as well as my team partners on that effort—Stuart Card, Peter Pirolli, and Mark Stefik from the Palo Alto Research Center (PARC) and John Bodnar from SAIC—for discussions and research that led to significant insights on current practices of analysis. I must again thank Paul Johnson and CSI for providing the opportunity to publish this study and reach a far broader audience; without that spur, I would not have completed it. And to the CSI editors, Mike Schneider and Andres Vaart, my appreciation for their great help in getting me through this entire process and in substantially improving this monograph.

Beyond those I have already mentioned, I am also truly obligated to a large number of busy people who took the time and made the serious effort to read and review the earlier briefing and draft study, as well as to share their perspectives and thoughts. Their comments and suggestions were crucial to producing what I hope is a coherent structure and argument: Art Kleiner, Dan Cohen, Jeffrey Pfeffer, Charles Sabel, Dick Kerr, Stephen Marrin, Bill Nolte, Harry Rowen, Mike Mears, Bruce Berkowitz, Mike Warner, Deborah Barger, Joe Hayes, Bill Studeman, Russ Swenson, Ed Waltz, Frank Hughes, Carol Dumaine, David Moore, Rob Johnston, Mark Lowenthal, Kevin O'Connell, Carmen Medina, Jim Bruce, Joe Keogh, Greg Giles, Winsor Whiton, Bob Cronin, Gilman Louie, and John Seely Brown. In addition, many thanks are due Emily Levasseur, my former research assistant, for her invaluable contribution in helping me to conduct the research, find important sources and citations, review thousands of pages of source materials, organize and edit, and revise numerous drafts—all in good humor.

Finally, I give my sincerest apologies if I have forgotten anyone who contributed time and effort to this project. For any errors of omission or commission, I have only myself to hold responsible.

About the Author

Jeffrey R. Cooper is Vice President for Technology, Chief Scientist of Strategies, and Director of the Center for Information Strategy and Policy at Science Applications International Corporation. He has undergraduate and graduate degrees from The Johns Hopkins University, where he was later Professorial Lecturer in Arms Control and Defense Analysis at the School of Advanced International Studies.

Mr. Cooper's core interest has been the use of information to improve intelligence analysis, decisionmaking, command and control, and operational effectiveness. During the past several years, Mr. Cooper has focused on analyzing intelligence failure and evaluating methods to improve all-source analysis. He was a professional staff member of the Presidential Commission on Future Intelligence Capabilities (The Silberman-Robb Commission).

With a long-time focus on strategic analysis and military transformation, Mr. Cooper is a founding member of the Highlands Forum, a program sponsored by the Secretary of Defense to identify national security-related cutting-edge technology. He has also served on numerous Defense Science Board task forces and summer studies. He has held senior government positions in the White House and the Department of Energy.

INTRODUCTION

As a result of a number of analytic projects for different intelligence agencies, a major focus of my work during the past several years has involved examining the practice of analysis within the US Intelligence Community.[1] This study was prompted by a growing conviction—shared by others, to be sure—that improving the analytic products delivered by Intelligence Community components had to begin with a critical and thorough appraisal of the way those products are created. A conversation with a physicist friend in 2002 had triggered thoughts on several basic differences between the practice of science and intelligence analysis. Shortly thereafter, an invitation to give a seminar on intelligence analysis at Stanford University led me to prepare a briefing entitled "Intelligence and Warning: Analytic Pathologies," which focused on a diagnosis of the problems highlighted by recent intelligence failures.[2] As Donald Stokes noted in his seminal book on science and technological innovation, *Pasteur's Quadrant*, "Pathologies have proved to be both a continuing source of insight into the system's normal functioning and a motive for extending basic knowledge."[3]

The Analytic Pathologies framework yields four insights that are crucial both to accurate diagnosis and to developing effective remedies. First, the framework enables analysts to identify individual analytic impediments and determine their sources. Second, it prompts analysts to detect the systemic pathologies that result from closely-coupled networks and to find the linkages among the individual impediments. Third, it demonstrates that each of these networks, and thus each systemic pathology, usually spans multiple levels within the hierarchy of the Intelligence Community. Fourth, the framework highlights the need to treat both the systemic pathologies and the individual impediments by focusing effective remedial measures on the right target and at the appropriate level. In response to presentations to community audiences, a number of senior intelligence officials subsequently recommended that I use the diagnostic framework of the briefing to develop corrective measures for the dysfunctional analysis practices identified there. I circulated the resulting draft for comment and was delighted to receive many useful suggestions, most of which have been incorporated in this version. Several knowledgeable readers of the draft also raised the issue of the intended audience, strongly suggesting that this should be the senior decisionmakers, in both the Executive Branch and Congress, who could take action to implement the ideas it presented. They also pointedly recommended that the study be substantially condensed, as it was too long and "too rich" for that readership. That audience is, after all, composed of very busy people.

From the beginning, however, I have intended this study to serve as a vehicle for an in-depth discussion of what I believe to be the real sources of the analytic pathologies identified in the briefing—the ingrained habits and practices of the Intelligence Community's analytic corps—and not the organizational structures and directive authorities that are the focus of most legislative and executive branch reformers. Thus, my intended audience has been the cadre of professional intelligence officers who are the makers and keepers of the analytic culture. Without their agreement on causes and corrective measures, I believe real transformation of intelligence analysis will not occur. Moreover, during the writing of this study, I was fortunate enough to serve on the selection panel for the inaugural Galileo Awards.[4] One of the winning papers focused on a similar issue—the appropriate audience for intelligence—and this reinforced my original inclination.[5] I have decided, therefore, not to condense this study in an effort to fit the time constraints of very high-level readers. I hope, instead, that the summary that follows this introduction proves sufficiently interesting to tempt them to tackle the remainder of the study, where the logic chains that I believe are necessary to convince intelligence professionals of the correctness of the diagnosis and the appropriateness of the suggested remedies are laid out in detail.

End Notes

[1] Although this paper will use the common terminology of "Intelligence Community" (IC), it is worth noting that the agencies of which it is composed seldom exhibit the social cohesion or sense of purpose that a real community should. A more appropriate term might be "intelligence enterprise," which is defined in Webster's Third International edition as "a unit of economic or business organization or activity."

[2] The briefing was first presented in early November 2003 to a seminar at Stanford University's Center for International Security and Cooperation (CISAC) and was revised for a Potomac Institute seminar on the "Revolution in Intelligence Affairs" on 17 May 2004. It will be cited hereafter as "Analytic Pathologies Briefing."

[3] Donald E. Stokes, *Pasteur's Quadrant: Basic Science and Technological Innovation.*

[4] The Galileo Awards were an initiative of DCI George Tenet, who, in June 2004, invited members of the Intelligence Community to submit unclassified papers dealing with all aspects of the future of US intelligence. DCI Porter Goss presented the first awards in February 2005.

[5] David Rozak, et al., "Redefining the First Customer: Transforming Intelligence Through Peer-Reviewed Publications."

SUMMARY

OBSERVATIONS

A wide range of problems has contributed to the unease currently pervading the Intelligence Community;[1] a significant number of the most serious result from shortcomings in intelligence analysis rather than from defects in collection, organization, or management.[2] The obvious and very public failures exemplified by the surprise attacks of 11 September 2001 and by the flawed National Intelligence Estimate (NIE) of 2002 on Iraqi weapons of mass destruction (WMD) have resulted in a series of investigations and reports that have attempted to identify the causes of those failures and to recommend corrective actions.[3] These recommendations have usually emphasized the need for significant modifications in the organizational structure of the Intelligence Community and for substantial enhancements of centralized authorities in order to better control and coordinate the priorities and funding of community entities. The Intelligence Reform and Terrorism Prevention Act (IRTPA) of 2004, which created the office of Director of National Intelligence (DNI), was based on such foundations.[4]

The logic of this study differs from most of those recommendations with respect to both causes and corrective measures. The key observations in the original "Analytic Pathologies" briefing point in a fundamentally different direction for the root causes of the failures and for fixing the manifest problems. Most importantly, these observations lead to the conclusion that the serious shortcomings—with particular focus on analytic failures—stem from dysfunctional behaviors and practices *within* the individual agencies and are not likely to be remedied either by structural changes in the organization of the community as a whole or by increased authorities for centralized community managers. Those key observations, which follow, provide the conceptual foundation for this study.

1. There Has Been a Series of Serious Strategic Intelligence Failures

Intelligence support to military operations (SMO) has been reasonably successful in meeting the challenges on the tactical battlefield of locating, identifying, and targeting adversary units for main force engagements. Similar progress in supporting counterterrorism operations has been claimed.[5] At the same time, however, other military and national users have been far less well served by the Intelligence Community across a range of functions. There have been significant shortfalls in support to post-conflict security and stabilization operations and reconstruction efforts in Iraq. Analytic support has also come up short both in accurately capturing adversary thinking and intentions and in providing intelligence that identifies and characterizes developing strategic challenges, such as WMD.[6]

Moreover, within the past decade and a half, a series of intelligence failures at the strategic level, including serious failures in operational and strategic warning, have highlighted real weaknesses at this level and undercut the confidence of principal national users in the community's capabilities against important intelligence targets. These failures include Iraqi WMD developments (1991 onward), the global black-market in WMD, strategic terrorism (beginning with the attack on the World Trade Center in 1993), the North Korean nuclear program (1994), the emergence of globally-networked Islamic fundamentalism (1996 onward), the Indian and Pakistani nuclear programs (1998),[7] the 9/11 attacks (2001), and Iran's WMD programs (2002). Similar failures, as well as an apparent inability to provide accurate assessments and estimates on other important issues, such as the nuclear forces and strategies of China and Russia, affect national users at the highest levels and outweigh any increases in effectiveness at the tactical level.

Indeed, as a bottom-line assessment, this study contends that the Intelligence Community has been least successful in serving the key users and meeting the primary purposes for which the central intelligence coordinating apparatus was created under the National Security Act of 1947.[8] These principal officials are the president and his cadre of senior national security policymakers, not the departmental and battlefield users. As a senior intelligence official recently reminded us, those objectives were two-fold: not only to provide "strategic warning" in order to prevent another surprise such as Pearl Harbor, but also to help head off long-term challenges through a better understanding of the emerging strategic environment.[9]

2. These Failures Each Have Particular Causes, but the Numerous Individual Problems Are Interrelated

These failures did not have a single locus—they occurred in technical collection, human source reporting, and analysis, among other critical functions—but neither do they reflect a series of discrete, idiosyncratic problems. Instead, they resulted from deep-seated, closely-linked, interrelated "systemic pathologies" that have prevented the Intelligence Community from providing effective analytic support to national users, especially effective anticipatory intelligence and warning.[10] The Intelligence Community's complicated organizational structure and the accreted practices of its analysts have combined to create what Charles Perrow calls "error-inducing systems" that cannot even recognize, much less correct their own errors.[11]

3. The Intelligence Community Still Relies on the Same Collection Paradigm Created for "Denied Areas"

Remote technical collection and targeted human access were appropriate means of penetrating denied areas and obtaining critical intelligence against a bureaucratized, centralized, and rigid superpower adversary that exhibited strongly patterned behavior. The problem presented by many of the new threats, whether from transnational terrorist groups or from non-traditional nation-state adversaries, however, is not that of accessing denied areas but of penetrating "denied minds"—and not just those of a few recognized leaders, but of groups, social networks, and entire cultures. Unfortunately, information for intelligence is still treated within the old "hierarchy of privilege" that emphasized "secrets" and was more appropriate for a bureaucratized superpower adversary who threatened us with large military forces and advanced weapons systems.[12] Without refocusing its energies, the Intelligence Community will continue to do better against things than against people.

4. Analytic Methods Also Have Not Been Updated from Those Used to Fight the Cold War

There were intelligence failures during the Cold War, but the United States and its allies managed to stay on top of the challenge presented by our principal adversary. A relatively stable threat (and consistent single target) allowed the Intelligence Community to foster in-depth expertise by exploiting a very dense information environment, much of which the opponent himself created. That "Industrial Age" intelligence production model—organized for efficiency in high-volume operations and fed by large-scale, focused, multiple-source collection efforts conducted mostly with episodic "snapshot" remote systems that were very good at big fixed targets—built a solid foundation of evidence. This knowledge base allowed analysts to cross-check and corroborate individual pieces of evidence, make judgments consistent with the highest professional standards, and appreciate and communicate any uncertainties (both in evidence and inference) to users. In particular, this dense information fabric allowed analysts to place sensitive intelligence gathered from human sources or by technical means within a stable context that enabled confirmation or disconfirmation of individual reports. As national security challenges evolved during the years following the collapse of the Soviet Union, however, continued reliance on the Cold War intelligence paradigm permitted serious analytic shortfalls to develop.

5. The Intelligence Community Presently Lacks Many of the Scientific Community's Self-Correcting Features

Among the most significant of these features are the creative tension between "evidence-based" experimentalists and hypothesis-based theoreticians, a strong tradition of "investigator-initiated" research, real "horizontal" peer review, and "proof" by independent replication.[13] Moreover, neither the community as a whole nor its individual analysts usually possess the ingrained habits of systematic self-examination, including conducting "after action reviews" as part of a continual lessons-learned process, necessary to appreciate the changes required to fix existing problems or to address new challenges.[14]

6. Intelligence Analysis Remains a "Craft Culture," Operating within a Guild Structure and Relying on an Apprenticeship Model That It Cannot Sustain[15]

Like a guild, each intelligence discipline recruits its own members, trains them in its particular craft, and inculcates in them its rituals and arcana. These guilds cooperate, but they remain distinct entities. Such a culture builds pragmatically on practices that were successful in the past, but it lacks the strong formal epistemology of a true discipline and remains reliant on the transmission, often implicit, of expertise and domain knowledge from experts to novices. Unfortunately, the US Intelligence Community has too few experts—either analytic "masters" or journeymen—left in the ranks of working analysts to properly instruct and mentor the new apprentices in either practice or values.

Conclusion

The Intelligence Community is not normally self-reflective and usually avoids deep self-examination, but recognition and acceptance of the seriousness of its problems by all levels of the community is a necessary prerequisite for true change, including significant modifications to current organizational cultures and ethos. Agreement on the basic diagnosis must, therefore, precede detailed propositions about effective remedies. I suggest that the following six premises, first articulated in the "Analytic Pathologies" briefing, summarize the most important conclusions to be drawn from the preceding discussion of the current enfeebled state of the Intelligence Community.

1. The Dysfunctional Practices and Processes That Have Evolved within the Culture of Intelligence Analysis Go Well Beyond the Classic Impediments Highlighted by Richards Heuer in the Psychology of Intelligence Analysis[16]

A more effective analytic paradigm must be built that incorporates the best analytic methods from modern cognitive science and employs useful and easily usable supporting tools to overcome these impediments and prevent them from combining into systemic pathologies.

2. More Corrosively, the Individual Impediments Form Interrelated, Tightly-Linked, Amplifying Networks That Result in Extremely Dysfunctional Analytic Pathologies and Pervasive Failure

A thorough reconceptualization of the overall analysis process itself is needed. The new approach would incorporate a better connected, more interactive, and more collaborative series of networks of intelligence producers and users.

In addition, it must be designed to detect and correct errors within routine procedures, instead of leaving them to be found by post-dissemination review.

3. The New Problems and Circumstances Call for Fundamentally Different Approaches in Both Collection and Analysis, as Well as in the Processing and Dissemination Practices and Procedures That Support Them

It is clear that serious problems in the existing organizational structure of the Intelligence Community are reflected in poor prioritization, direction, and coordination of critical collection and analysis activities.

However, many problems that are more fundamental and deep-seated exist inside the organizational "boxes" and within the component elements of the intelligence agencies themselves.

Fixing these—dysfunctional processes, ineffective methods, and ingrained cultures—is not solely a matter of increased authorities, tighter budgetary control, or better management.

A strategic vision that addresses the systemic pathologies, leadership that understands how key functions ought to be improved, and a sustained long-term commitment to rebuilding professional expertise and ethos will be essential.

4. Accurate Diagnosis of the Root Causes of Problems "Inside the Boxes" Is Required; Otherwise Remedies Will Be Merely "Band-Aids"

For example, the analytic problems occur at and among four organizational levels: 1) individual analysts; 2) analytic units, including their processes, practices, and cultures; 3) the individual intelligence agencies; and 4) the overall national security apparatus, which includes the entire Intelligence Community in addition to the executive bodies responsible for making policy. Solving problems at all four of these interlocking levels requires an integrated attack that includes solutions addressed to the right level and tailored for each problem element.

5. The Intelligence Community Must Bring More Perspectives to Bear on Its Work and Create More Effective "Proof" and Validation Methods in Constructing Its Knowledge

It should, in particular, adopt proven practices from science, law, and medicine, including more open communication and self-reflection.

6. Whatever the Details of Structures or Authorities, the New Director of National Intelligence (DNI) Leadership Must Assure That the Corrective Measures Are Implemented within Each Agency and Across the Community

Moreover, all this should be done in the knowledge that change will be continual and that there will be no static resting place where the "right" solutions have been found; organizational structures and processes must be designed to evolve with and adapt to that realization.[17]

Recommendations

Curing the flaws in intelligence analysis will require a sustained emphasis on rebuilding analytic capabilities, refocusing on human cognitive strengths enhanced by innovative support tools, and restoring professional standards and ethos among the analysts themselves. Most of the recent reform recommendations notwithstanding, more guidelines and tighter management oversight are no substitute for analytic expertise, deep understanding, and self-imposed professional discipline—all achieved not only by formal education and training, but also through assimilation from following experienced mentors. Moreover, neither curiosity nor expertise on the part of the individual analysts can be restored by directives from the top; they must come from an appropriate recruiting profile, effective training, continual mentoring at all levels, time to learn and practice the craft of analysis— both individually and collaboratively—and constraining the "tyranny of the taskings" that prevents analysts from exercising curiosity and pondering more than the obvious answer.[18] To ensure that the Intelligence Community can provide more effective capabilities to meet the increasingly complex challenges of 21st-century security issues, this study recommends rebuilding the overall paradigm of intelligence analysis from its foundations. The essential components of this effort are:

1) A revamped analytic process;
2) An entirely revised process for recruiting, educating, training, and ensuring the professional development of analysts (including the essential aspect of mentoring);
3) Effective mechanisms for interactions between intelligence analysts and users;
4) A proper process for "proof," validation, and review of analytic products and services;
5) An institutionalized lessons-learned process;
6) Meaningful processes for collaboration within the Intelligence Community.

Furthermore, although implementing each of these processes separately would produce significant improvements in the quality of analysis, a more effective approach would be to mount a broad-gauged, systematic, and integrated effort to deal with the entire analysis process.

End Notes

[1] See The 9/11 Commission Report: Final Report of the National Commission on Terrorist Attacks Upon the United States (cited as the 9/11 Commission Report) and Report on the

U.S. Intelligence Community's Prewar Intelligence Assessments on Iraq by the US Senate Select Committee on Intelligence, 7 July 2004 (hereinafter cited as SSCI Report).

2 See Henry A. Kissinger, "Better Intelligence Reform," Washington Post, 16 August 2004: 17.

3 For a review of the various commissions that have tackled intelligence reform, see Michael Warner and J. Kenneth McDonald, US Intelligence Community Reform Studies Since 1947. A detailed look at the work of one such recent commission is Loch K. Johnson, "The Aspin-Brown Intelligence Inquiry: Behind the Closed Doors of a Blue Ribbon Commission," Studies in Intelligence 48, no. 3 (2004): 1– 20. Still, there is no guarantee that good intelligence will necessarily help decisionmakers reach good judgments or make good decisions, but poor intelligence can clearly corrupt good decision processes and amplify ill-advised tendencies in flawed processes.

4 Intelligence Reform and Terrorism Prevention Act, PL 108–458, 2004 (hereinafter cited as IRTPA).

5 See Testimony by Cofer Black, Coordinator for Counterterrorism, US Department of State, before the House International Relations Committee, 19 August 2004.

6 It appears, for example, that the intelligence needed to support the security and stabilization operations in Iraq with effective "cultural awareness" during the post-conflict "Phase IV" has been far less than adequate. See comments by senior military officers at a conference in Charlottesville, Virginia, sponsored by CIA's Center for the Study of Intelligence (CSI). Intelligence for a New Era in American Foreign Policy, (hereinafter cited as Charlottesville Conference Report), 3–5.

7 Perhaps the more serious error in the case of the Indian-Pakistani nuclear tests was not the failure to predict the timing of the catalytic Indian test (which was really more a failure by policymakers); arguably, it was the failure to estimate correctly the scale and status of the Pakistani weapons program, including its links to the global WMD black market.

8 Michael Warner, "Transformation and Intelligence Liaison," SAIS Review of International Affairs (hereinafter SAIS Review) 24, no. 1 (Winter-Spring 2004): 77–89

9 See Deborah Barger, "It is Time to Transform, Not Reform, U.S. Intelligence," SAIS Review 24, no. 1 (Winter-Spring 2004): 26–27.

10 The systemic pathologies are discussed in detail in Chapter Three.

11 Charles Perrow, as cited in Robert Jervis, "What's Wrong with the Intelligence Process?" International Journal of Intelligence and Counterintelligence 1, no. 1 (1986): 41. See also Charles Perrow, Normal Accidents: Living with High-Risk Technologies.

12 Fulton Armstrong, "Ways to Make Analysis Relevant But Not Prescriptive," Studies in Intelligence 46, no. 3 (2002): 20.

13 "Evidenced-based" analysis is essentially inductive; "hypothesis-based" is deductive; they should be seen as complementary approaches, not competitors for ownership of the analytic process.

14 For an exception, see John Bodnar, Warning Analysis for the Information Age: Rethinking the Intelligence Process. In fact, both the Joint Military Intelligence College (JMIC) and the Center for the Study of Intelligence have programs to create a discipline of intelligence by bringing together intelligence theory and practice. Regrettably, the results of these efforts have not yet penetrated the mainline analytic units.

15 In fact, the analytic community self-consciously characterizes its practices and procedures as "tradecraft."

16 Richards J. Heuer Jr., The Psychology of Intelligence Analysis. Building on the work on cognitive impediments to human judgment and decisionmaking of Daniel Kahneman, Amos Tversky, and others, in addition to his own long experience as a senior intelligence analyst,

Heuer highlighted many psychological hindrances to making accurate judgments by individuals and small-groups.

[17] A medical analogy might make this argument clearer. Although a low-cholesterol diet, proper exercise, routine physicals, a low dose of aspirin, and moderate intake of alcohol may be useful over the long-term for preventing heart disease, patients in acute cardiac distress require more forceful intervention to save them. The measures listed above would have been useful before the attack, and they may be appropriate after recovery, but they are not effective during an acute crisis or in the immediate aftermath, when patients must be kept under observation to be certain they are "taking their medicine."

[18] Professor Jeffrey Pfeffer of the Graduate School of Business at Stanford University is one of several commentators who have emphasized the importance of "slack" to enable collaboration and collective efforts—including discussion, review and comment, professional development, and service to the "community of practice," as well as pursuing the scent of curiosity.

Chapter 1

Making Sense of the US Intelligence Community

A Complex Adaptive System

With its fifteen diverse agencies and its wide range of functional responsibilities, the Intelligence Community presents a very complicated set of organizational arrangements. Thinking of it in terms of traditional organizational analysis or systems engineering methods in an effort to explain its working does not suffice because it far more resembles a living ecology with a complex web of many interacting entities, dynamic relationships, non-linear feedback loops (often only partially recognized), and specific functional niches that reflect momentarily successful adaptations to the environment.[1] These complex interrelationships among its components create dynamic adaptations to changing conditions and pressures and make the Intelligence Community especially difficult to understand.[2] In fact, it is an exemplar, even if not a healthy one, of a truly complex adaptive system.

During the Cold War, proportionately more resources supporting a larger cadre of experienced analysts devoted to a simpler and relatively static priority target, as well as a broad array of established sources, disguised many of the Intelligence Community's dysfunctional aspects and growing internal problems. The community's loosely federated structure and complicated, if not Byzantine, processes had previously appeared tolerable, even if not fully successful, because making changes appeared to present a greater risk.[3] In the face of a drastically changed security environment, however, it is exactly the combination of complexity and opaqueness that has masked the increasingly dysfunctional misalignment of "dinosaur" analytic processes and methodologies from earlier recognition by both analysts and consumers of intelligence, much less by outsiders.[4]

> The Intelligence Community is an exemplar, even if not a healthy one, of a truly complex adaptive system.

Even for insiders, the workings of the Intelligence Community are difficult to understand because, as a rule, its members are not deeply self-reflective about its practices and processes. For outsiders, however, these difficulties are magnified by the community's compartmentation, security restrictions, and intrinsic opaqueness. That is why applying traditional organizational analysis that concentrates on structure is doomed to failure; understanding these complex adaptive systems requires more synthesis than traditional "reductionist" analysis.[5] In this case, moreover, it is a complex adaptive system that, insulated by security barriers, has managed to ignore and—probably because of its centralized direction, however imperfect—suppress important external signs of change and to amplify self-protective internal signals, which often reflect strongly ingrained cultural preferences.

The results of the Intelligence Community's failure to recognize the increasing dysfunction were both paradoxical and unfortunate. They were paradoxical because—although it has been accused of not adapting to dramatically changed conditions—the community adapted all too well. And they were unfortunate because the pressures to which it did adapt flowed from misperceptions inside and outside the Intelligence Community engendered by the collapse of the Soviet Union: that there would be no significant challenges to American interests; that the end of the Cold War reduced the need for a "national security state"; that there should be a substantial "peace dividend," a large part of which would be paid by the Intelligence Community. The community's adaptive processes did accommodate these changes internally—especially the need to "survive" the huge budget cuts and to become relevant to the articulated needs of the paying customers.

> It is important not only to locate the level at which obvious symptoms occur, but also the level at which problems can be solved.

However, these internal pressures outweighed the huge new challenges emerging in the external security environment. Responding to these would demand new expertise and a new knowledge base, along with appropriate methods, tools, and perspectives—all of which required more resources, focused leadership, and strong commitment, which was not there. As a result, the community fostered a series of processes that were increasingly mal-adapted to needs emerging in the new geostrategic environment. By responding to the wrong signals, it created Perrow's "error-inducing systems."[6]

Relating Structure and Process

Unfortunately, most Intelligence Community reform proposals concentrate on changes in structure and in directive and managerial authorities. Analytic problems, however, actually take place not just at the level of the community as a whole, but at four distinct levels, as well as in the complex interrelationships, both vertical and horizontal, among them.[7] Thus, it is important not only to locate the level at which the obvious symptoms appear, but also the level at which the problem can be solved. In this way, the root causes of failure can be identified and appropriate and effective corrective measures taken.

The National Security Community

The relevant entities include the National Security Council (NSC), the Office of the Director of National Intelligence (ODNI), and the national policymaking and operational elements in the Department of State and the Department of Defense.[8] Among the failures at this level can be misdirected priorities and misallocation of resources; poor communication and coordination; and inconsistent apportionment of authority, responsibility, and capability among the main entities. Such failures flow downward and can easily percolate throughout the subordinate organizations. For the Intelligence Community, a particular problem at this level may involve its relationships with top-level users, especially managing their expectations. On the one hand, for example, the Intelligence Community often demonstrates an inability or unwillingness to say "no" to consumer requests, which leads to additional priority taskings without concomitant resources or relief from other ongoing activities. Similarly, the Intelligence Community often conveys an illusion of omniscience that fails to make clear its state of knowledge on an issue, the underlying quality of the intelligence, or the degree of uncertainty—all of which can leave the Intelligence Community seemingly responsible for decisions taken on the basis of "bad intelligence."

The Intelligence Community

This level currently includes the fifteen component intelligence agencies. Failures at this level can include misdirected priorities and budgetary allocations within the Intelligence Community; lack of effective procedures and oversight of them among component agencies; poor communication and coordination among agencies; a lack of enforceable quality-control processes; toleration of substandard performance by individual agencies; poor communitywide technical standards and infrastructure that hinder information sharing; and poor management and oversight of security procedures that impede effective performance. Errors at this level also encompass failures by groups or individuals to make critical decisions, to exercise appropriate authority, or to take responsibility for gross errors that should be worthy of sanction or dismissal.[9]

The Individual Analytic Units and Organizations

It is essential to appreciate the importance of particular analytic environments within specific sub-organizations— an office within the CIA's Directorate of Intelligence, for example. It is these entities, rather than the organization as a whole, that create the work processes and practices that form the immediate cultural matrix for an analyst's behavior.[10] Failures at this level can include dysfunctional organizational processes, practices, and cultures that inhibit effective analysis by individuals and sub-units; management attitudes and directives that stress parochial agency objectives; toleration of poor performance; excessive compartmentation and special security procedures that erect barriers to effective execution; poor prioritization and assignment of workflow; inability to create and protect "slack" and conceptual space for intellectual discovery; ineffective recruitment and training; maintaining stand-alone information and analysis infrastructures, including ineffective support for individual analysts; poor direction and management of the analytic process; and, simply, ineffective management of the analytic cadre. This is probably the most important level for creating consistently high-quality analysis because of its impact on the analytic environment, on the selection of methods and processes, and on the work life of individual analysts. Errors at this level are perhaps the most pernicious, however, and they have been widespread and persistent.

Individual Analysts

Failures at this level can include poor performance due to lack of ability, lack of domain knowledge, lack of process expertise, poor social network contacts, or ineffective training; pressures to favor product over knowledge; lack of time; being too busy and too focused to maintain peripheral vision and curiosity, even on high priority work; failure to cooperate and collaborate with others; lack of suitable tools and support; misguided incentives and rewards; and an organizational culture and work practices that tolerate second-rate analysis. To illustrate the impact of this multi-level hierarchy and underscore the importance of correctly identifying the locations of causative factors in analytic errors, for example, consider the case of an analyst who fails to interpret correctly the evidence pertinent to a task and draws a wrong conclusion. At first glance, the obvious approach should be to focus corrective actions on the analyst: what caused the failure, and what are the appropriate remedies? Simple incompetence, a rush to complete the assignment, a lack of domain knowledge needed to recognize critical linkages, or a failure to employ appropriate methods could all be causative factors. At this level, the obvious remedies to these problems are better screening, training, and mentoring.

It could be, however, that the problem lies with the analytic unit, its work processes, and its management: the tasking was high priority, and this analyst, whose expertise is on another subject, was the only one available; appropriate tools and methods were not provided; training in relevant domain knowledge or on effective new tools had been postponed due to production pressures; or, given the production cycle, the analyst lacked sufficient time to search for all the relevant evidence. The problem could reside even farther up the hierarchy, among the agencies of the Intelligence Community: key data from another agency was not made available, due to compartmentation restrictions or because incompatible information infrastructures prevented the analyst from easily searching another agency's holdings. Finally, the failure could actually reside at the topmost level, with community management: this account was given such low priority that no collection resources had been assigned to gather information or to provide consistent analytic coverage or, because of the thinness of the evidence base, the inability to answer the question was not made clear to the requester at the start. However, it is exactly here that the "5 Whys Approach" of the Quality Movement proves its value.[11] Applying this approach, which features a progressively deeper, recursive search, forces the investigator to trace a causative factor to its source.[12] Assume that, in this example, it is a lack of domain knowledge.

> Why was an analyst not fully knowledgeable in the domain working that account?
> She was covering for the lead analyst, who is away on temporary duty (TDY).
> Why did the analytic manager assign that analyst to the task?
> She was the only one available.
> Why was the analyst not fully knowledgeable on her backup account?
> She is an apprentice analyst with only a short time on the account and inadequate mentoring. Her training had been postponed due to scheduling. She didn't have time to be curious and follow the information scent. She could not access the lead analyst's "shoe-box."[13]
> Why couldn't she access the shoebox of the lead analyst?
> It is his personal collection of tentative hypotheses and uncorrelated data kept as a personal Word file and is not in an accessible database. The shoe-box is actually a pile of paper put in temporary storage when the lead analyst went on TDY.
> Why is the lead analyst unwilling to share his shoebox?
> Why is there no accessible collaborative system for sharing shoeboxes?

The questions would continue through as many rounds as the questioner needed to satisfy himself that he had found the root cause.

Although the previously cited reports on intelligence failures usually point to organizational stove-piping and technical shortcomings as the most important contributors to failures in collaboration, the sources of such failure are actually more widespread and complex—and more frequently reflect shortcomings in work practices and processes, organizational culture, and social networks.[14] In addition, the proposed solutions that focus on structures and authorities disregard the critical interrelationship between structure and processes and ignore as well the importance of organizational culture on institutional effectiveness. As Stephen Marrin, among others, has noted:

Structure and process must work together in a complementary fashion, and structural changes alone without corresponding changes to existing processes would simplify the workings of the Intelligence Community in some ways, but cause greater complexity in others.[15]

The significant structural reforms legislated in 2004 will also entail substantial short-term transition costs to effectiveness as new organizational arrangements are implemented, processes are developed, and outmoded roles and systems are replaced. The really difficult task will be to redesign the processes, so that they are consistent and complementary to the structural changes that are being made.

Incorrect diagnoses of the causes of analytic failures probably arise from not recognizing the variety and complexity of the roles, missions, and tasks that confront analysts.

The Analysis Phase-Space

At a basic level, incorrect diagnoses of the causes of analytic failures probably arise from not recognizing the variety and complexity of the roles, missions, and tasks that confront analysts.

This diversity results in a complex phase-space that contains a significant number of discrete analytic regions. These certainly cannot be treated as though their perspectives and needs were homogeneous or even similar. The tasks required of a signals intelligence analyst attempting to locate a terrorist's cell-phone call are fundamentally different from those of an all-source analyst drafting an NIE on Chinese strategic nuclear doctrine. Therefore, because intelligence collection and analysis are not based either on a suite of all-purpose tools or on fungible human expertise that can be instantly swiveled to focus effectively on a different set of problems, this phase-space also implies the need for a similar diversity of analytic processes, methods, knowledge bases, and expertise.

Differentiating Intelligence Roles

Moreover, given this diverse phase-space, conflating three distinct roles played by all-source intelligence adds to the underlying confusion over intelligence missions and functions, the priorities among them, their requirements, and the capabilities needed to make each effective. The traditional assumption that there were only two sets of intelligence consumers, each with distinct mission needs, often led to contraposing support to military operations, which was assumed to be tactical in focus, and national user support, which was assumed to demand deep analysis. In reality, meeting the disparate needs of the users intelligence must serve requires recognizing three distinct roles for all-source intelligence.[16] Two of them, Support to Military Operations (SMO) and Support to Policy Operations (SPO), focus primarily on issues needing immediate information capabilities to assist decisionmaking on current operations. Although SMO and SPO issues are of interest to both national and departmental users, the third role, Warning and Estimative Intelligence (WEI), largely emphasizes issues that are almost exclusively the province of national users and usually take place over longer time horizons.[17]

In all cases, however, although it still uses the term "support," the Intelligence Community must move beyond the notion that it is segregated from the rest of the national security community and that it merely provides apolitical information to decisionmakers. Intelligence has now become an integral element of both the policy and military operational processes; and the success or failure of its judgments can have the most significant consequences in both domains.[18] Increasingly-integrated military operations, in which intelligence directly drives operations, and command centers in which intelligence personnel are fully integrated, are tangible evidence of such changes. As a result, it is important that intelligence appreciate not only the centrality of its role, but also the increased obligations and responsibilities that such a role brings.[19]

Support to Military Operations (SMO)

This traditional intelligence role has usually focused on assisting current military operations. Much of this information concerns current numbers, locations, and activities of hostile units, and other information addresses significant elements of the physical environment in which military forces are operating.[20] Other military users need quite specific current data on subtle technical characteristics of adversarial equipment and forces to serve, for example, as targeting signatures or to support electronic warfare (EW) activities. Regardless of type, intelligence supporting operating forces demands extraordinary accuracy, precision, and timeliness to ensure that it is immediately "actionable" under conditions that are highly stressful and potentially lethal.[21]

Increasingly, however, military operators have other operational intelligence needs, such as support for information operations and for security and stabilization in Iraq. To prosecute these missions successfully, the military now also needs far more cultural awareness and timely accurate information on adversary thinking, motivations, and intentions.

Support to Policy Operations (SPO)

Making explicit that this is a distinct role emphasizes the importance of intelligence to daily policymaking across the entire spectrum of national security concerns; it is the "national user" cognate of SMO. SPO provides policymakers and senior officials (importantly including senior civilian defense officials, combatant commanders, and other military officers) with indispensable situational awareness, including important background information, to assist them in executing and overseeing ongoing policy activities and in planning and framing policy initiatives. As it is as intensely focused on providing actionable information, it is as heavily oriented as SMO to current intelligence and reporting. However, SPO differs from SMO somewhat in content and priorities in that it has always included a greater proportion of less quantifiable, softer information, such as political and economic trends in major countries and groups and assessments of foreign leaders and their intentions.

> A warning process ... allows decisionmakers to think through responses they might be obliged to make in haste.

Warning and Estimative Intelligence (WEI)

Mary McCarthy, a former National Intelligence Officer (NIO) for Warning, commented on the recommendations of a DCIchartered study conducted in 1992:

> According to that ten-member panel of highly respected intelligence and policy veterans, providing policymakers with persuasive and timely intelligence warning is the most important service the Intelligence Community can perform for the security of the United States.[22]

McCarthy defines warning as "a process of communicating judgments about threats to US security or policy interests to decisionmakers."[23] Thus, warning provides vital support to "national users" in their principal *strategic* missions—understanding the complex geostrategic environment, fostering vision of objectives, assessing alternatives and determining strategy, and protecting against consequential surprise; most importantly, when done properly, warning is forward looking and anticipatory.[24]

Warning is sometimes thought to be merely alerting decisionmakers to immediately threatening activities, but, in reality, it is a far more complex function and actually addresses two very different kinds of problems. One type of warning is concerned with monitoring activities previously recognized as potentially dangerous, such as a hostile missile launch, and cueing appropriate responses. The second type is a discovery function that assists decisionmakers in identifying those situations and activities whose consequences could have significant (and usually adverse) effects—and which may not necessarily be obvious. When performed effectively, a warning process provides decisionmakers with an anticipatory sensitization that allows them to think through, in a disciplined way, the responses they might someday be obliged to make in haste. Assessments and estimates, on the other hand, also are usually forward looking, but they are designed to be informative rather than part of a process closely tied to triggering contingent responses.

Further complicating the matter is that both types of warning also operate over three different horizons. *Strategic* warning has always been understood as looking out toward the distant future; it is intended to recognize that a possible threat may be looming—even if it is not imminent—and to provide time to take appropriate preparatory actions, including policies and actions that might prevent the threat from eventuating.[25] *Operational* warning also looks out in order to identify the characteristics of the threat (the likely and particular methods of attack), so that offsetting contingency plans and actions can be prepared. From this detailed understanding of enemy intentions, capabilities, and concepts, operational warning also serves to identify indicators that an attack is in preparation. Finally, *tactical* warning is the immediate alerting function that a specific (with respect to time, place, or character) hostile activity has begun or is about to begin.

An important but often overlooked element of warning over all three horizons is the key role played by negative evidence, which can help confirm that potentially threatening activities are **not** occurring and prevent costly and potentially consequential responses from being taken or scarce resources from being squandered.[26] During the confrontation between the United States and the Soviet Union, and, in particular, during periods of high tension between them, one of the most important functions of warning was to inform the leaders that, "Today is not the day."

Both the warning and estimative functions are designed to focus more on informing decisionmaking with context and long-term implications than with supporting ongoing activities. The preparation of assessments and estimates, as well as development of warning indicators, has more to do with analysis and judgment than with reporting; it demands deep expertise as well as an ability to place knowledge of the subject in broad context. These important functions serve the entire national security community.[27]

Although warning is often misconstrued as a current intelligence problem, even tactical warning of specific targets, times, and means must build on this deeper foundation of pre-emptive analysis of threats and responses if it is to be effective. During the Cold War, recognizing that we were engaged in a long-term competition, we were prepared to adjust our intelligence priorities so that analysts could provide assessments of future capabilities and indications of intentions, even though the day-to-day threats were most grave. As was the case in facing the Soviet Union, there may well be tensions today in choosing between serving SMO and SPO, on the one hand, and assuring adequate resources for WEI, on the other hand, as continued access to information needed for an understanding of enemy intentions and capabilities could be sacrificed by meeting the needs for immediately actionable intelligence.

Today's decision-makers have many more sources of information than did their predecessors... ; in turn, the Intelligence Communityholds far less of a monopoly over information about foreign events and technology developments.

Although warning and estimative intelligence may be seen as the core missions of strategic intelligence, they are also less tied to the details of ongoing operations in which the formal relationships between policymakers and intelligence provide a unique advantage and leverage for intelligence insights. Today's decisionmakers have many more sources of information than did their predecessors when the Intelligence Community was created; in turn, the Intelligence Community holds far less of a monopoly over information about foreign events and technology developments. Moreover, as one senior intelligence official noted, policymakers see themselves and their staffs as substantively knowledgeable on issues of interest as the Intelligence Community and capable of serving as their own intelligence analysts.[28] As a result, users increasingly see themselves as participants in a process of judgments.[29] An experienced national-level user wrote recently,

> Today, the analyst no longer sets the pace of the information flow. The sources of information now available to the policy-level consumer...are far, far greater than a quarter century ago. It is almost a given that today's policy-level consumer of intelligence is well informed in his or her area of interest and not dependent on an intelligence analyst for a continuing stream of routine, updating information.[30]

IMPLICATIONS OF DIFFERENTIATING ROLES

Careful differentiation among the three intelligence roles discloses dimensions that are both analytically important and more meaningful for contemplating intelligence reform than the usually misleading bimodal distinctions between national vs. military users or tactical vs. strategic objectives. What truly distinguishes these intelligence roles is their *perspective and emphasis*—a significant distinction that has been lost in recent arguments over intelligence reform.

To begin with a particularly important point, a tactical or a strategic focus does not necessarily distinguish military from civilian users.[31] Moreover, the less quantifiable and, therefore, *softer* information and analysis on individuals, decisionmaking, and social dynamics that used to be produced primarily for national users is now increasingly demanded to support military operations at the tactical level. Such information is inherently more judgmental and inferential—and, therefore, less precise—than analysis of physical or technical characteristics in orders-of-battle (OOBs) and tables of organization and equipment (TOEs). It is less amenable to counting or to the gathering of external physical signatures by technical collection systems; it is more dependent on language skills, deep expertise on the region and cultures, and knowledge of the personalities.[32] It is also harder to validate or prove than estimates of technical factors. Such capabilities go beyond "reporting" that used to be the core of current intelligence.

However, both SMO and SPO are, by nature, mission- or task-oriented and tightly focused on the problem at hand; and this narrowed focus has significant time and perceptual implications for analysts and the intelligence sources supporting them.[33] Given the stress, time pressures, and immediate—as opposed to potential—stakes attendant on current operations, human decisionmakers try to concentrate only on the immediate situation and the information relevant to it, while actively screening out other inputs. This is the intelligence analogue of human "foveal vision," which offers the highest visual resolution but also a very narrow field-of-view.[34]

In contrast, warning and estimative intelligence are the analogues of human "peripheral vision," in which there is low resolution but a wide field-of-view. Peripheral vision is very sensitive to cues of dynamic change, which trigger anticipatory responses. Although warning is concerned with activating the response cycle, and estimative intelligence is intended to create a frame of reference for the decisionmaker, both are intended, through preconditioning and anticipatory consideration, to enable a more appropriately and contextually sensitized response on the part of users.[35]

Another important implication of the differing emphasis on decisions with a long-term view and those requiring prompt action— the classic distinction between strategic and tactical—concerns the nature of the advantage to be gained from the information, and, therefore, how it is exploited. In recent years, the tasks of intelligence, and its successes and failures, have focused on providing immediately actionable (in this sense, tactical) intelligence to users—information that can provide a rapid or near-instantaneous advantage, whether for interdicting hostile military forces, preventing terrorist incidents, or supporting diplomatic initiatives. Emphasizing current intelligence for actionable exploitation may have created an unintended mind-set that undervalues the immense importance of knowing and understanding the adversary's intentions throughout the course of the confrontation, even at the cost of foregoing exploitation of these sources for temporary advantage on the battlefield or in the diplomatic conference room.[36] This stress on current intelligence also influences the priorities among the types and attributes of information we collect, the nature of the collection and processing systems, the analytical methods we use, the stresses we place on analysts, and the metrics by which we assess the performance of intelligence.[37]

There is yet another important distinction between these roles. By looking out to the future, WEI is basically a surprise-preventing function intended to heighten a policymaker's ability to visualize the consequences of anticipated and unanticipated events and to prepare for them mentally; it is not designed to be "evidence-based truth-telling" that will stand up in court. In addition, as we better appreciate the implications of emergence and the emergent behaviors of complex adaptive systems, we need to place greater emphasis on anticipation while recognizing that precise prediction or forecasting is even harder than previously understood. Appreciating the differences in perspective created by these roles is very important because failing to make clear distinctions between them may aggravate a major problem before the Intelligence Community: the disconnect between the emphasis on current reporting or providing situational awareness, which must be evidence-based, and the policymaker's need for anticipatory judgments, which, by nature, trade the confidence derived from hard evidence for an intuitive, or *gestalt,* understanding of the whole derived from inference.[38] It is unlikely that analysts will have firm evidence to offer the policymaker to support alternative interpretations of the future, and they will need to rely on inference and informed speculation that is persuasive to decisionmakers.[39] In particular, as one experienced intelligence analyst noted,

> "Getting inside the other guy's head" can only be conjectural because, in most cases, even the "other guy" doesn't know exactly why he's doing what he's doing.[40]

Even if there are predictive judgments to be made in both SMO and SPO,[41] they tend to have short time horizons and reasonably short inferential chains; as the predictive time-constants are short, observation of adversary actions can serve to validate or disprove these judgments and thereby improve confidence in them and the analyst's judgment.

> When one tries to assess the adequacy of Intelligence Community performance ... or prescribe changes ... the appropriate answers will almost certainly differ greatly from one role to the other.

Those providing SPO, in particular, must continually walk a fine line between serving the policymakers' needs for relevant, focused, direct support and maintaining objectivity in providing the evidence and analysis. Staying close to the evidence assists the analyst in walking this line. At the same time, the author of this monograph noted a clear consensus among senior intelligence officers at a recent non-attribution conference that analysts can best serve policymakers by offering them thoughtful and thought-provoking views that challenge their assumptions. It must be recognized, however, that helping to alter policymakers' assumptions is intruding directly into the policymaking process and, thereby, crossing the boundary that Sherman Kent tried to establish. As the policymakers demand judgments on actions and consequences farther in the future (moving the intelligence role from SPO to WEI), not only will the intrinsic uncertainties increase, but also the potential for tensions between policymaker and analyst over the objectivity (and validity) of the judgments and the conflicts among differing judgments.[42]

Another of these distinctions affects intelligence requirements and planning. Unlike SMO and SPO, where the users can clearly identify their areas of interest, priority issues, and information needs, the Intelligence Community must look beyond its users' perceptual horizons if it is to perform warning and estimative functions effectively. Almost by definition, with anticipatory intelligence, policymakers will be unable to tell the community where to look. Unfortunately, although the Intelligence Community must recognize that attempting to divine requirements for warning and other anticipatory intelligence from the users is not likely to be fruitful, it also must appreciate that it alone will bear the blame for failing to warn against the inevitable surprises arising from outside the fields-of-view of users. This demands, in turn, that the Intelligence Community have some discretion and flexibility to allocate resources in areas not currently considered to be priority targets: listening too closely to the customers, and looking only where directed, guarantees future strategic warning failures.

It is absolutely essential that the Intelligence Community and those who depend on it understand the principal distinctions between these two functions. In their conclusions about the nature of the Intelligence Community's problems, the extraordinary differences between the report of the 9/11 Commission and that of the SSCI on Iraqi WMD reveal the dangers of conflating the two distinct functions or ignoring the differences between the three roles. When one tries to assess the adequacy of Intelligence Community performance across these domains, identify shortfalls, or prescribe changes—whether in business practices, tools, or organizational arrangements—the appropriate answers will almost certainly differ greatly from one role to the other.

End Notes

[1] A feedback loop, in systems analysis, is a relationship in which information about the response of the system to stimuli is used to modify the input signal (see "Feedback," *Principia Cybernetica Web*). A non-linear loop is one that creates non-proportional responses to stimuli.

[2] See Peter M. Senge, *The Fifth Discipline: The Art & Practice of the Learning Organization*. Senge is the founder of the Organizational Learning Laboratory at MIT.

[3] The pressures of the Manichean confrontation with the Soviet Union tempered enthusiasm for drastic and disruptive changes. These might have improved effectiveness, but they would also have provoked bureaucratic and congressional battles over power and jurisdiction.

[4] After all, the dinosaurs were superbly adapted to their environment; even if they perceived the signals of change, they became extinct because they could not adapt to unfamiliar environmental conditions.

[5] An appreciation of the distinction between a complicated system and one that is complex and adaptive is important for accurate diagnosis and effective solutions. A hallmark of complex adaptive systems is that they produce "emergent behavior," which cannot be prediced by analysis of their component elements or structure.

[6] See Perrow, *Normal Accidents.*

[7] The briefing on "Analytic Pathologies" describes the multi-level interplay of these problems. See Appendix A for a summary.

[8] At this level, for the Intelligence Community, it is the ODNI and the Intelligence Community elements that are responsible for critical functions—collection, analysis, special activities, and community management—that interact directly with senior principals. With a DNI and an ODNI organization in place, these relationships are likely to become even more complicated.

[9] See Statement by Admiral David Jeremiah (USN, ret.), Press Conference, CIA Headquarters, 2 Jun 1998, for a suggestion that failures by senior managers to make key decisions had been an important factor in the CIA's failure to warn of an impending Indian nuclear test. (The subject was the "Jeremiah Report" on the 1998 Indian nuclear test.)

[10] See Karl E. Weick, *Sensemaking in Organizations*.

[11] The Quality Movement took root in the United States during the 1990s, when US auto manufacturers were challenged by the emergence of higher quality Japanese automobiles made by automakers who had adopted the principles of two US engineers, W. Edwards Deming and Joseph Juran. The principles provide a systematic set of processes and metrics for improving the quality of manufacturing processes.

[12] A recursive search is one in which successive searches build on the results of earlier searches to refine the answers returned. (See National Institute of Standards and Technology, *Dictionary of Algorithms and Data Structures*.)

[13] Although seldom used today, many analysts once referred to the personal files where they stored such items as the results of research as "shoeboxes." It is used here to emphasize the particularity of the methods employed by analysts.

[14] Technical systems and infrastructures enabling collaboration are important, but they are only a small part of the solution to fostering effective collaboration. For more on this topic, see discussion beginning on page 57.

[15] Stephen Marrin, in a review of William E. Odom, "Fixing Intelligence: For a More Secure America," *Political Science Quarterly*, 119, no. 2 (Summer 2004): 363.

[16] It is important to recognize that these regions have fuzzy boundaries, overlap to some degree, and are not totally distinct.

[17] The intelligence role that often leads to confusion over appropriate categorization is warning, and especially the tactical warning component. Because warning is intimately connected to a decision on a responsive action, it is sometime mistakenly considered to be a decision-support activity; in reality, it is more appropriately seen as a part of the informative function that assists policymakers in thinking about issues before they occur, helping to create coherent, contextualized reference frames. Moreover, because tactical warning is *tactical*, it is often forgotten that it is of principal concern to high-level strategic users because it

almost always involves activities that could have the most serious political and strategic consequences. Thus, these three roles cover two distinct functions: SMO and SPO emphasize situational awareness and immediate decision support, while WEI focuses on anticipation of future circumstances.

[18] I am grateful to Dr. Russell Swenson of the Joint Military Intelligence College for persuading me to sharpen this point. See Russell G. Swenson, with Susana C. Lemozy, "Politicization and Persuasion: Balancing Evolution and Devolution in Strategic Intelligence," unpublished manuscript. When the CIA was created, expectations about intelligence capabilities and its role were significantly different than they are today. At the policy level as well, there is now an expectation that intelligence will be available to guide policy creation and inform course changes if necessary.

[19] A valuable guide to appropriate comportment in these circumstances is Herbert Goldhamer's *The Adviser.*

[20] The US Army, which has extensive doctrine on operations, calls this intelligence preparation of the battlefield (IPB). This includes specific information on mission, enemy, time, terrain, and troops available (METT-T).

[21] A critical example is the need for technical details, so that enemy weapons, such as improvised explosive devices (IEDs), can be countered.

[22] Mary McCarthy, "The National Warning System: Striving for an Elusive Goal," *Defense Intelligence Journal* 3 (1994): 5. Warning is considered the classic "strategic intelligence" role and was the principal reason for the creation of the CIA.

[23] Ibid.

[24] There have always been terminological problems associated with the word "strategic." During the Cold War, users of the word often conflated level of analysis (global and synoptic), time horizon (forward-looking), and magnitude of the stakes (very large), with instrumentality (nuclear) and distance (intercontinental).

[25] To some degree, these terms have always been confusing because they described two very different types of problems. Strategic, operational, and tactical warning related to surprise nuclear attack were very patterned, but focused on two distinct problems: surprise attack executed by known forces and surprises that were truly unanticipated.

[26] Perhaps the scarcest resource is a senior decisionmaker's attention, which can easily be wasted.

[27] As an indication of the long time horizon involved in this function, both civilian and military defense officials need to look well into the future to develop strategy, plan forces, support research and development, and acquire systems.

[28] See Charles E. Allen, "Intelligence: Cult, Craft, or Business?" in "Comments of the Associate Director of Central Intelligence for Collection" at a Public Seminar on Intelligence at Harvard University, spring 2000. See http://pirp. harvard.edu/pdf-blurb.asp?id+518: 15. Henry Kissinger may be the most obvious example of this tendency, but it has continued since the Nixon administration and has come to include a far greater proportion of policy officials, especially as the sources of information on foreign developments have expanded dramatically and become available in near real-time. See Henry A. Kissinger, "America's Assignment," *Newsweek*, November 8, 2004: 38–43.

[29] As one senior intelligence official remarked in a private meeting, "We are all in the business of making judgments; but too many in the Intelligence Community continue to believe that they are instead providing crystalline analyses."

[30] Clift, "Intelligence in the Internet Era," *Studies in Intelligence* 47, no. 3 (2003).

[31] This distinction might have been clearer before civilian leaders began taking detailed interest in overseeing tactical operations—as began during the Vietnam War with presidential interest

in the selection of bombing targets. With respect to the Soviet Union during the Cold War, national and military users had clear areas of primary interest; national users were focused on intelligence illuminating key political, economic, technological, and social factors affecting national power and intentions, while military users were more focused on the likely force capabilities and doctrines of potential adversaries. After the Cold War, improving technical capabilities and the emergence of the "strategic corporal" combined to increase the interest of civilian policymakers in overseeing tactical operations.

[32] Several senior military participants at the Charlottesville conference highlighted these demands. See *Charlottesville Conference Report*, 2–5.

[33] There is a very large body of literature on the physical and psycho-perceptual effects on human judgment and decisionmaking under stress that is relevant to these distinctions.

[34] The fovea, a small pit at the back of the retina, forms the point of sharpest vision. The intensely narrow concentration of foveal vision is recognized as being a major contributor to "change blindness."

[35] One type of warning function amenable to focused monitoring involves potential surprise from a recognized adversary undertaking a feared but pre-identified activity (such as a Warsaw Pact invasion across the Inner-German border). This other warning function serves to guard against truly unexpected or unforeseen events. In both cases, they are designed to encourage thinking about, and contingency planning for, "surprises" before they occur.

[36] The widely repeated—but apocryphal—story that perhaps best exemplifies this understanding of "strategic intelligence" is that of Churchill's allowing Coventry to be bombed in order to safeguard the long-term informational advantages gained from Allied code-breaking achievements against the Axis. The immeasurable importance of such intelligence in the successful Allied efforts to interdict Rommel's supply lines during the North African campaign and in winning the crucial Battle of the Atlantic testify to these other equities with possibly higher priority.

[37] Barger, 26. Although her specific comment refers to the impact of precision (timeliness and resolution, for example) on the quality and quantity of intelligence, her larger point is that functional needs stemming from roles and missions drive what the Intelligence Community provides its users and how it does so.

[38] *Gestalt*, a German word meaning "form" or "shape" is used in psychology to connote holistic understanding of the entirety of a phenomenon. This follows Kendall's approach of "creating pictures," as noted by Jack Davis in "The Kent-Kendall Debate of 1949," *Studies in Intelligence* 35, no. 2 (1991).

[39] This is a comment to the author by a senior intelligence officer who has served in both roles.

[40] Private communication to the author from John Bodnar, 3 November 2004.

[41] The military, in particular, is increasingly emphasizing "predictive battlespace intelligence" as a central component of "information superiority." It is usually, however, a different kind of prediction than that required to support SPO.

[42] As the founder of Air Force and Joint Staff Studies and Analyses, Lt. Gen. Glenn Kent (USAF, ret.), paraphrasing Shakespeare, once warned analysts, "Neither a prostitute nor a proselytizer be."

Chapter 2

ASSESSING CRITICAL ANALYTICAL SHORTFALLS

As astute members of the Intelligence Community have observed, intelligence capabilities (and the organizations that provide them) are not general purpose tools but, rather, specialized and "finely honed" instruments that evolve and adapt to the specific challenges and requirements placed upon them.[1] Many of today's principal analytic problems arise from continued reliance on analytic tools, methodologies, and processes that were appropriate to the static and hierarchical nature of the Soviet threat during the Cold War and were, in that environment, largely successful. We possessed several decided advantages that enabled us to overcome some of the limitations on our capabilities: a careful and cautious "Main Enemy" that was also a far simpler and slower target than those we face today; more time; many and more experienced analysts; and varied and well-established sources of information, including the adversary's own vast outpouring of seemingly trivial but very useful data.

Given these advantages, the Intelligence Community was able to:

- Concentrate, focus, and build a deep foundation of cumulative evidence;
- Foster longstanding and deep expertise in its analytic cadre by exploiting a very dense information environment;
- Rely on multiple-source collection, which generally allowed us to cross-check information and make judgments consistent with the highest professional standards;

- Largely neglect intelligence collection and analysis on "soft" cultural, societal, and people issues (other than the most prominent elites), because the plans and intent of the adversary were in the hands of a small Politburo and because we "knew" that knowledge of the plans and intent of subordinate elements or nations—for example, Poland—was rarely necessary;[2] and
- Employ an intelligence model that could rely on collecting "secrets" in voluminous quantities and required a mass production approach for producing reports.[3]

That was also a period of relative information scarcity on worldwide events, and the Intelligence Community had a substantial comparative advantage over other information providers through access to intelligence obtained by clandestine collection.

The United States had many Cold War successes, of course, but there were always significant shortcomings in American intelligence capabilities. These shortcomings resulted in surprises that had important and unanticipated consequences for US policy. Among these were the Egyptian/Syrian attacks on Israel opening the 1973 Yom Kippur War, the 1974 Indian nuclear test, the fall of the Shah and the accompanying ascendance of a fundamentalist Islamic regime in Iran in 1979, the unexpectedly rapid collapse of the Warsaw Pact in 1989, and the dissolution of the Soviet Union in 1991.

> Many of today's principal analytic problems arise from continued reliance on analytic tools, methodologies, and processes that were appropriate to ... the Cold War.

The traditional intelligence methods were even less successful against some important targets that have carried over into the post-Cold War era—such as Iran, China, North Korea, nuclear proliferation, and the global WMD black-market. In these cases (exemplified by the 1998 Indian and Pakistani nuclear tests), we have had serious shortcomings in understanding because, in the face of the numerous, continuing, and competing demands for higher priority current intelligence, we were unwilling or unable to make the long-term commitments to build the deep knowledge base the task required.

Today, the United States may need to take action more frequently on the basis of ambiguous intelligence, against harder to recognize threats, from less risk-averse enemies—especially the shifting groups of radical Islamic fundamentalists who foment terrorist activities and may wield capabilities that could devastate cities, societies, or economies. These new Islamic adversaries also pose, as did the Soviet Union, a longterm ideological challenge whose character and "operational code" we do not currently understand. Unlike the Soviet Union, however, which was a hierarchical, bureaucratic state whose organizational character we did understand, the new targets are more dynamic and complex. These new groups morph frequently and metastasize like cancers, emerging with new personalities and network linkages and threatening new targets.[4]

As a result, today's Intelligence Community must contend with:

- Little foundational knowledge on major adversaries and cultures;
- Fragmentary evidence and sparse intelligence flows, which often cannot be substantiated or contextualized—even against the highest priority current targets;
- Thin domain ("account") expertise, due to multiple and shifting priorities and frequent shuffling of relatively inexperienced analysts;[5] and
- An analysis model that remains heavily dependent on "secrets," even when the key intelligence questions may involve mostly "mysteries" and "obscurities."[6]

Aggravating these existing shortcomings, a cascade of significant and complex developments that will pose substantial new challenges is already evident, making the adequacy of the community's current capabilities even more problematic.[7] These changes involve more dynamic geostrategic conditions, more numerous areas and issues of concern, smaller and more agile adversaries, more focus on their intentions and plans and less on large physical objects and weapons systems, a more open information environment, and more widespread understanding of American intelligence methods and capabilities by our adversaries. Additionally, the sense of vulnerability to terrorist attack on US territory left by 9/11 has created huge new demands on the Intelligence Community to provide information for homeland security.[8] The immensity of these challenges complicates the task of developing appropriate cures for the real causes of inherited shortcomings and of heading off new analytic shortcomings.

The lengthy reports of the 9/11 Commission and the SSCI report on Iraqi WMD laid out in great detail their views on why these two failures occurred. Although they occurred in very different substantive domains, at very different levels of analysis, in different parts of the intelligence organizations, and exhibited significantly different failure modes and causative reasons, both reports tended to locate the causes in problems related to information sharing and coordination, instances of insufficient collection and poor data, and "errors" of analytic judgment by individuals and groups.[9]

The Intelligence Community now finds itself under intense scrutiny and faced with the need to transform in fundamental ways in order to meet the entire range of national security intelligence challenges only partially recognized in the legislatively mandated reforms. Addressing these challenges requires fundamentally new approaches in both collection and analysis as well as in the processing and dissemination methods that support them. As Barger aptly notes: what is needed is revolution, not reform.[10]

MISUNDERSTANDING ANALYTIC PROCESSES

The litany of failures should have been a tip-off to the deep-seated nature of the analytic problems. Such a series of "idiosyncratic" errors by individuals and small groups within an organization are, however, more likely to be symptoms than root causes, as Perrow convincingly demonstrated in case studies of Three Mile Island and Chernobyl.[11] A pattern of repeated errors is often a signal of seriously dysfunctional methods—fundamental and systematic failures of procedures and processes throughout an organization.[12] From this perspective, the proximate causes of the failures identified in both the report of the 9/11 Commission and the SSCI report on Iraqi WMD hardly appear to be convincing root causes of these recent intelligence failures.

> Major American corporations have fallen victim to a pattern of "overadaptation" and "change blindness." The Intelligence Community runs the same risk.

A more accurate diagnosis of the sources of our intelligence shortcomings requires a deeper and more thoughtful analysis of why organizations make mistakes—causes that go beyond obvious superficial conditions created by flawed organizational structures and insufficient directive authorities. As Charles Sabel noted, "There he [Herbert Simon in *Administrative Behavior*] showed that modern organizations were efficient precisely because they systematically turned habits—the disposition to react to particular situations in a characteristic, but open-ended way—into rigid routines."[13] Not unexpectedly, these routines "work" for the specific conditions they were developed to address. They rarely perform well for off-design conditions, however, and, often, the better they work for the design conditions, the more narrow the set of conditions for which they are appropriate. Paradoxically, the better they work, and, therefore, the more efficient the organization at its routine tasks, the greater the danger that the organization will fail to be sensitive to its environment and changes occurring there. As with the dinosaurs, scores of major American corporations have fallen victim to this pattern of "over adaptation" and "change blindness."[14] The Intelligence Community runs the same risk.

Talk of a "science of analysis" is a conceit… . The reality is otherwise.

The Problem of the Wrong Puzzle

Frequent public references to "failing to connect the dots" are especially problematic for an accurate understanding of intelligence errors and failures. This view of the analytic shortfalls is particularly perverse, because it masks the true nature of the analyst's challenges. The flawed "connect the dots" analogy flows from the image of the children's game book in which lines are to be drawn between a set of numbered dots in order to make a recognizable picture. That analogy assumes, however, that—as in the children's book—the dots exist, that it will be obvious which dots connect to which others and in what order.[15] The problem is that this simple analogy overlooks a well-known phenomenon in psychology that is often illustrated by the "Rubin Vase Illusion": that evidence really does not "speak for itself"; rather, that information is "perceived and interpreted."[16] Humans are extremely good at finding patterns, even when there is none—hence the classic intelligence aphorism, "You rarely find what you're not looking for and usually do find what you are looking for."[17]

If we are to use a puzzle analogy, perhaps a more appropriate model might be that of a guest at a resort hotel who, on a rainy afternoon, wanders into the game room and finds a box holding a large number of jigsaw puzzle pieces. As the cover of the box is missing, there is no picture to guide him in reconstructing the puzzle, nor is there any assurance that all the pieces are there. Indeed, when he discovers that there are several other empty puzzle boxes on a shelf, it is not even clear that all the pieces in the box belong to the same puzzle. Reconstructing the puzzle in this example is a far different and more difficult challenge than linking numbered dots, where the outline of the image is reasonably apparent.[18]

Both the dots analogy and the model of evidence-based analysis (discussed in the following section) understate significantly the need for imagination and curiosity on the part of the analyst.

THE MYTH OF "SCIENTIFIC METHODOLOGY"

Many well-informed outside commentators and intelligence professionals continue to talk about the "science of analysis," and only some of them are truly aware of the shaky foundations of this belief or of its real implications.[19] But this talk of a "science of analysis" is a conceit, partly engendered by Sherman Kent's dominating view of intelligence analysis as a counterpart of the scientific method.[20] The reality is otherwise; analysis falls far short of being a "scientific method" in the common, but usually misunderstood, sense. Moreover, this view of science itself is "scientism," which fails to recognize the important role of less "rational" and less "scientific" elements, such as imagination and intuition.[21] As Mark and Barbara Stefik, knowledgeable and respected participants in the discipline of science, have written about science and innovation in a recent book.

> The word "theory" usually connotes a formal way of thinking logically or mathematically. In this formal sense, theory takes its place in a knowledge-generating process called the scientific method. The scientific method includes hypothesis formation, experiment planning, execution, and data analysis. In this scheme, theory is used to make predictions. Theory is created by a process that includes hypothesis formation and testing.
>
> Unfortunately, this notion of theory and the working methods of science and invention leaves out imagination. This makes it both boring and misleading....[22]

Citing a well-known commentary by a Nobel laureate, the Stefiks add:

> In [Peter] Medawar's view, the standard scientific paper promotes an error of understanding how science is done because it confuses proving with discovering.[23] The layout of a scientific paper makes it appear that the doing of science is the careful laying out of facts. Once the facts are in, the conclusions follow. This makes it seem like science is all about deduction. Unfortunately, this formal structure leaves out the creative part

of discovery and invention. The structure of a scientific paper is only about proof, promoting the systematic marshalling of evidence. In this abbreviated story, once a scientist has by some means figured it out, the paper lays out the conclusions logically.[24]

A more realistic and useful appraisal of the process of intelligence analysis comes from Charles Allen, a long-time senior intelligence official: "I want to speak mainly about the art and craft of intelligence.... We could have talked about the science of intelligence, but, by and large, as far as I'm concerned, the science of intelligence is yet to be invented. I don't see it. It's not really there."[25] This is not to suggest that rigor, accuracy, clarity, and precision are not required in intelligence analysis; given the stakes, they are obviously essential. But demanding a false precision from an analysis process that is itself incorrectly modeled on a common misunderstanding of the methods of science is not likely to improve the quality of analysis. Indeed, an important issue for both managers and users of analysis to consider is the likelihood that there may be little concordance between precision in the details of the answer and the accuracy of the overall *(gestalt)* judgment. A process and methodology too focused on provable evidence may get the details right at the cost of ignoring important inferential judgments that need to be conveyed in order to provide a true sense of the uncertainties of both evidence and judgment.[26]

> A process and methodology too focused on provable evidence may get the details right at the cost of ignoring important inferential judgments.

THE FLAWS OF A "TRADECRAFT" CULTURE

Intelligence analysis remains largely a craft culture that is conducted within a self-protective guild system and taught by means of a broken apprenticeship process. There are other fields, such as science, medicine, and warfare, in which knowledge is also understood to be tentative and not subject to formal "proof," as is possible in mathematics. Within such professions, the cumulative practices, habits, and mindsets of an evolved culture are especially important for the creation of knowledge and the transmission of expertise. As with intelligence, these other communities are ones in which much of the knowledge needed for effective performance relates to the often-arcane processes of the craft (tradecraft, as the Intelligence Community terms it). This knowledge is tacit and difficult to elicit from the experts, and it is usually best communicated by personal example and practice.[27] However, the culture of intelligence lacks many of the formalized processes, such as "peer review," and the cumulative knowledge structures that the academic, military, and medical communities have created to address similar challenges in building a solid foundation of understanding that can be passed to successor practitioners. Perhaps for these reasons, intelligence analysis is not yet a true profession. Within this culture, therefore, effective mentorship is especially important for transmitting expertise and, perhaps more significantly, for imparting professional standards and values to apprentices.

End Notes

1 See Aris A. Pappas and James M. Simon Jr., "The Intelligence Community: 2001–2015," *Studies in Intelligence* 46, no. 1: 39–47; Bruce Berkowitz, "Intelligence for the Homeland," *SAIS Review* 24, no. 1 (Winter-Spring 2004): 3.

2 To appreciate the costs of this view, see the brief account on page 41 of Professor Murray Feshbach's use of Soviet and Russian health statistics to derive an important conclusion.

3 The bureaucratized nature of the Soviet Union and the state of telecommunications throughout the Cold War allowed the United States to exploit its technological prowess and employ effective remote collection capabilities in addition to the traditional method of using human sources.

4 Marc Sageman, "Understanding Terror Networks," FPRI E-Note, 1 November 2004.

5 In addition, inexperienced analysts may lack the ability to tap sources of deep expertise available through connections to long-standing professional networks.

6 Fritz Ermarth originally developed this typology. For the details, see page 40.

7 Barger, 28.

8 At the same time, the breaching of old distinctions between foreign and domestic intelligence activities has increased public concern over potential threats to privacy.

9 Indeed, the IRTPA was largely driven by the recommendations of the 9/11 Commission, which focused mostly on one, albeit important, aspect of intelligence needs, that of counterterrorism. But, as noted above, the IRTPA reforms mandate changes that affect all functions of the Intelligence Community.

10 Barger, 28.

11 Perrow, *Normal Accidents*.

12 For examples of the consistent nature of such errors, see the following: the "Jeremiah Report"; Interview with Richard Kerr, MSNBC, 14 July, 2003 (concerning the "Kerr Report" on the Iraqi WMD NIE). An unclassified portion of that report is in *Studies in Intelligence* 49, no. 3 (2005) (hereinafter cited as Kerr, et al.).

13 Charles F. Sabel, "Theory of a Real Time Revolution."

14 See Carol Loomis, "Dinosaurs?" *Fortune*, 3 May 1993: 36*ff.* An accompanying sidebar recounted how a senior Sears executive pointed behind himself to the tens of volumes of corporate practices and rules that governed the corporate response to any conceivable problem. The emergence of mid-market national discount chains wasn't covered; and, therefore, "...wasn't a problem they had to address."

[15] This relatively simple problem is known formally in mathematics as a "directed graph."

[16] Edgar Rubin, 1915. Heuer discusses such perceptual problems using different examples in Chapter 2 of *The Psychology of Intelligence Analysis*.

[17] This remark is often attributed to Amrom Katz, a pioneer in aerial and overhead reconnaissance.

[18] Heuer, Chapter 6.

[19] See, for example, Frank Hughes and David Schum, *Evidence Marshalling and Argument Construction*.

[20] Sherman Kent, *Strategic Intelligence.* See also Jack Davis, "The Kent-Kendall Debate."

[21] The term "scientism" is used to connote the frequent confusion between the appearance of a formal scientific methodology and the actual conduct of science, which may be intuitive, but is nonetheless subject to rigorous proof.

[22] Mark Stefik and Barbara Stefik, *Breakthrough: Stories and Strategies of Radical Innovation*, 110.

[23] The Stefiks are referring to Peter Medawar's article, "Is the Scientific Paper Fraudulent? Yes; It Misrepresents Scientific Thought," published in the *Saturday Review* 47, 1 August 1964: 42–43.

[24] Stefik and Stefik, 110–11.

[25] Allen.

[26] For more on this subject, see the section on "Evidence-based Scientism" in Chapter Three.

[27] The professions of medicine and law refer to themselves as "practices," which reflects their roots in the guild system. More importantly, perhaps, this usage conveys that the essential elements of a profession (ethos, ethics, and skills) are human values best transmitted by people.

Chapter 3

AN INVENTORY OF ANALYTIC PATHOLOGIES

Although many of the reform proposals responding to the recent intelligence failures took diametrically opposed positions with respect to the role of the DCI, the creation of the DNI, and the functions of the CIA within a "transformed" Intelligence Community, they were mostly quite similar in that they focused both on wiring diagrams and formal authorities as the mechanisms for reform and on creating a "czar" to execute those authorities through centralized management.[1] As is often the case, reform legislation took a structural route to address problems that flow from dysfunctional processes, inbred cultural practices and habits, and failures of human leadership.

> ... establishing more centers with mandated institutional positions and priorities can only further dilute an already overstressed cadre of intelligence professionals.

Although the legislative changes have restructured the community, other than emphasizing "competitive analysis" and more HUMINT, the IRTPA contains little significant language about reforming the internal functional processes of intelligence— collection and analysis. The legislation failed to take into account several key distinctions that any intelligence reform proposals must recognize: differences in issue domains; tactical vs. strategic consequences; narrowly focused vs. synoptic collection and analysis; reporting vs. deep analysis; immediate vs. long-term decision horizons; foveal vs. peripheral perception; action vs. exploitation; and defined, tasked requirements vs. speculative information gathering.

Some recommendations, in fact, could aggravate the already dysfunctional conditions, further damaging analytic capabilities. The IRTPA directed the establishment of centers for priority issues, as recommended by the 9/11 Report, but these are likely to place even more emphasis on current intelligence, whether or not this was intended. Integrated centers combining operators and analysts do foster better sharing and collaboration among them, but they invariably place the emphasis for analysts on operational support. Moreover, creating static structures and rigid processes designed to deal with fixed areas or issues is not a particularly sound response to events and conditions that are very fluid and fuzzy. These can be better handled by operating within a process that allows flexibility and discretion. Finally, with an already severe shortage of effective managers and experienced intelligence officers (including analysts, operators, and collectors), establishing more centers with mandated institutional positions and priorities can only further dilute an already over-stressed cadre of intelligence professionals.

An Inventory of Analytic Pathologies

Curing analytic shortcomings cannot be done by making minor modifications to the existing processes or even by wholesale replacement or upgrading of the analytic cadre.[2] Although it may be tempting to focus on better educating and training the analysts—the better for them to be able to "connect the dots"—altering the analytic model and the processes on which that model relies is almost certainly a more appropriate response to the profound problems besetting intelligence analysis. Without fixing the fundamental shortcomings in analytical processes, the system will always depend on the ability of individuals to work around the impediments, which adds additional stress to an already burdensome set of tasks.

At the same time, it should be acknowledged that there are limitations on the depth and quality of the expertise available within the community. The past decade has shown that the Intelligence Community is likely to find itself behind academic and commercial sectors in many frontier areas simply because, for the most part, that is where these frontiers are first explored. Furthermore, given the unpredictable nature of emerging challenges and the often short response time they allow, the community is unlikely to have on hand sufficient regional, cultural, linguistic, technical, or specialist expertise to meet high priority threats to our national interests. Therefore, unless community management decides to forgo having all needed expertise within the community—to open its boundaries, remove the barriers, and create mechanisms to draw on external expertise and knowledge—these impediments to exploiting outside expertise will frustrate its ability to meet emerging mission challenges.

Interestingly, even if the old analytic methods and processes developed during the Cold War were themselves capable of addressing the emerging security challenges of post-Soviet adversaries, a review of postmortems of intelligence failures prior to 9/11 and the Iraqi WMD fiasco showed that these processes and procedures were routinely violated, frequently leading to failures.[3] In addition to shortcomings in the basic analytic paradigm and processes, according to the study, the system lacked enforceable self-correcting features and functioning compliance mechanisms. This suggests that there has been a more fundamental failure in leadership and in the basic institutional and management mechanisms for assuring effective performance of oversight, assessment, accountability, and responsibility. That these failures persisted for so long should be of concern to members of the analytic community, their leadership and management, and the oversight bodies as well. It is a warning sign that better oversight and enforceable compliance procedures are needed, because the analytic community itself may no longer possess the internal self-discipline or professional standards to do so.[4] This also clearly implies that greater attention to professional ethos and standards must be an integral part of efforts to transform analysis.

Indeed, well before 9/11, several articles written by experienced community officials pinpointed fundamental shortcomings within the community's analytical capabilities and highlighted dysfunctional processes as the causes.[5] Thus, the longstanding failure modes within the existing intelligence analysis paradigm must be identified and corrected, along with the management and oversight procedures, if the community is to meet new needs.[6]

Two elements of the current paradigm are especially worthy of attention.

First Is the Inefficiency of the "Account" Structure

The account system, by its very nature, creates institutional and individual "ownership" of important intelligence domains. The benefit is that it provides a basis for accountability; the disadvantage is that ownership inhibits sharing, cooperation, and collaboration. It has also encouraged "stovepiping" by collection discipline and the control of information by collectors through originator-control (ORCON) restrictions. A fundamental redesign of analysis should start by dismantling both the notion of information ownership and the paradigm of "accounts," while maintaining accountability for performance; information must become the common property of the community, and someone with authority must oversee sharing and configuration management.[7] Such changes are likely to involve altering the existing institutional mechanisms in order to forge interagency virtual "clusters" to perform the analytic functions while creating "mission managers" with the authority to assure that important subjects and user needs are properly serviced.

A fundamental redesign of analysis should start by dismantling both the notion of information ownership and the paradigm of "accounts."

The Second Element Is the Intelligence Community's Strong Cultural Orientation Towards an "Evidence-Based Scientism"

Although this approach may be appropriate for the current intelligence functions that rely heavily on gisting and reporting and dominate both SPO and SMO, it clearly limits the ability of analysts to address the anticipatory intelligence needs of decisionmakers, which usually demand more reliance on judgments and inference chains and less on specific evidence. In return for more focus on the WEI role, decisionmakers who rely upon anticipatory intelligence must realize its inherent properties and limitations and be prepared to accept greater uncertainty in assessments and estimates in order to obtain better gestalt understanding.[8]

We need to understand that "warning" is largely built on modeling (either explicit or implicit) and synthesis, which are deductive processes, and not on analysis, which is an inductive process. In all cases, analysis processes should also access more non-traditional sources and incorporate a wider range of information to construct corroborative fabrics that can confirm or disconfirm critical information and hypotheses. The rigor and strength of these methods must rely less on narrow tests of the quality of the evidence or adherence to formalisms than on analysts being sufficiently "mindful" to recognize the pitfalls they may encounter in blind application of approved methodologies.[9] In addition, there is a huge research literature on decisionmaking under uncertainty that could be exploited to introduce innovative techniques for analysis and decision support. What all this comes down to, however, is not to disregard the need for rigor of method and quality of evidence, but, rather, to suggest that a construct of analysis too narrowly tied to a misunderstood "scientific method" needs to be augmented and leavened with intuition, curiosity, and a thirst for discovery—all essential elements of good science.[10]

Beyond these two fundamental changes, eight other problematic features of the current intelligence environment need to be addressed.

3. The Tyranny of Current Intelligence

Over the past decade, the Intelligence Community's efforts to be responsive to its customers' demands for current intelligence have dominated collection and analysis. As a senior analyst noted, "The Intelligence Community really [is] focused on current intelligence, on policy support. It does very little research. It has very little understanding below the level of the policymaker and, in my view, on many issues. I think that, in some ways, these two groups are reinforcing each other's worst habits."[11] The disappearance of the long-term Soviet threat and the chaos of the post-bipolar geostrategic environment shifted policymaker interests to a series of *crises du jour*. Policymakers demanded that intelligence for their current problems receive priority as the US and Allied interventions in Somalia, Haiti, Bosnia, Kosovo, and elsewhere proceeded. At the same time, the Pentagon's increasing demands for support in ongoing military operations, including such prolonged activities as *Northern* and *Southern Watch* in Iraq, placed tremendous demands on the intelligence system for a continuing stream of timely support products.[12]

Prior to the 1991 Gulf war, no commanders of regional or functional military forces— other than those for strategic forces—could expect to receive direct and timely support from national assets, especially to support tactical operations.[13] That war, and the glimpse it provided of the power of modern information systems to overcome shortcomings in C4ISR (command, control, communications, computers, intelligence, surveillance, and reconnaissance) fueled an intense push to obtain "information superiority." This, in turn, created nearly insatiable appetites among military commanders for real-time intelligence support and gave birth to the concept of "net-centric warfare" (NCW).[14] Many of the new C4ISR systems (including national systems), and much of the effort and funds expended by the Intelligence Community since the Gulf War, have focused on providing direct, real-time support to forces engaged in combat by closing the "sensor-to-shooter" loop and to meeting the information needs of the senior-level commanders directing those operations.

When there are American forces deployed in active military operations, as there have been on a near-continual basis since the end of the Cold War, the highest priority is now accorded to providing intelligence to support them.

4. Overemphasis on Production

At the same time as demands to support military operations generated huge requirements across the Intelligence Community, standing collection and analysis requirements to fill databases and to produce routine scheduled products set priorities for a substantial part of the intelligence "phase-space." The entire intelligence system is dominated by the demands of processing huge amounts of information gathered by collection systems whose architecture was largely designed during the Cold War to address a very different problem. This huge inflow created a production-oriented model and an "efficiency paradigm" better suited to the "Industrial Age" than to the Information Age of the Twenty-first century.[15] The volume of collected intelligence is so vast that, even with automated assistance, human analysts can effectively review and evaluate only a small part of the flow.

The existing paradigm for intelligence analysis and dissemination still relies largely on published paper reports as the mechanism for delivering products to users. Furthermore, without effective metrics to assess the value of intelligence to decisionmakers as well as the impact of analysis on the quality of their decisions, it is simple measures of data collected, traffic processed, and reports produced that have influenced critical decisions on priorities and resource allocation within the Intelligence Community. Meeting the new challenges will require a greater emphasis on adaptability and agility, as well as processes that are better able to respond to non-routine requests and high-priority challenges. The price to be paid for this, however, may be a reduction in efficiency as measured by the usual output-oriented metrics of mass-produced products normally used in cost-benefit calculations of routinized processes. Such calculations underweight the ability to meet unexpected situations and the "slack" that is usually essential in an adaptable organization.

5. Over-Reliance on Previous Judgments

The problem of "finished intelligence" stems from the conceit that any intelligence product is more than a snap-shot of knowledge believed to be true at that time and that "finished intelligence" is, by virtue of the formal coordination and review processes, "truer" than the pieces of raw intelligence from which it was built. The roots of this conceit date back to the period when the Intelligence Community was seen to possess domain expertise found neither in its user communities nor outside government, and its assessments could be considered authoritative. During that period, the Sherman Kent posture of standing apart from policy users could be considered an appropriate style. Fully coordinated "finished intelligence" products, such as NIEs, do convey authoritativeness as the *current, agreed judgment* of the Intelligence Community. These products also carry a sense that they and their conclusions can stand the test of time. These latter assumptions, however, are not necessarily warranted. As most "finished" intelligence products involve substantial interpretation, analysis, synthesis, and judgment, and they are more likely to have lengthy inference chains that compound uncertainty issues in more fragmentary reporting.

> The community too often treats probing questions as attempts to "shape" (that is, "politicize") analyses rather than genuine inquiries into the quality of evidence and the strength of inferences.

The validity of the earlier judgments expressed in finished products is especially important because of the common practice of "layering," that is, using previous, formally coordinated products as the starting point for new assessments and estimates.[16] Although this practice helps to assure the consistency of an analytic line, building on established judgments or on prior positions of an analyst, branch, group, office, or agency is also a reason to be wary. As a former senior intelligence official noted, *Judgments which any analytical actor has the greatest incentive to defend must be subjected to the most critical scrutiny.*[17]

The danger arises because, unlike academic practice, there is no sustained or sanctioned process of after-the-fact ("ex post facto" or "ex post") review. Finished products are rarely subjected to a considered re-examination, nor do they receive explicit testing by other parties trying to replicate their findings—unless there is an obvious major intelligence failure. Moreover, errors that are recognized subsequent to publication are often not corrected, by means either of timely notification to readers or of corrections fully incorporated throughout the knowledge base.[18] Other knowledge intensive enterprises, such as law, medicine, and science, also depend on cumulative foundational knowledge;

but they do far better at maintaining the accuracy and currency of these critical intellectual resources than does the Intelligence Community.

Even a cursory reading of the report on Iraqi WMD highlights the mutually reinforcing dangers of the “finished intelligence” conceit and of “layering.” Too often, the presumed authoritativeness of a formal product leads users to accept its judgments as established and its underlying evidence as validated. These products then become the baseline for updated assessments, and, as a result, the cumulative impact of errors is amplified and becomes pervasive.[19] In fact, the conceit is even more damaging to the effectiveness of the Intelligence Community in an era when policymakers are increasingly likely to be their own “senior analysts” and may not believe that “finished intelligence” represents the final word on a topic. Today, these officials bring other information and their own expertise to the task of arriving at a comprehensive judgment, and intelligence material is only one input into that process.[20] Yet the community too often treats probing questions as attempts to “shape” (that is, “politicize”) analyses rather than genuine inquiries into the quality of evidence and the strength of inference chains.

> Waiting on the policy community to furnish requirements for anticipatory intelligence all but assures that there will be serious warning failures.

6. The Neglect of Research

This emphasis on current intelligence, with its consequent time pressures and the methods needed to meet production demands, has produced a range of distorting effects that are not fully recognized.[21] First, it has severely undercut the ability of analysts to do in-depth research by requiring that most analytic effort be devoted to short-term taskings. Second, by denying most analysts the opportunity to work on deep products under the tutelage of a senior mentor, this emphasis has damaged a key element of the indispensable apprenticeship process, a *sine qua non* for effectively training and developing professionally competent intelligence practitioners. Third, in order to meet daily requirements, the production aspects of the current intelligence cycle have been accorded undue priority.[22] Fourth, the emphasis on current intelligence helped to create an incentives and rewards system for the analysts biased towards short-term reporting rather than deep analysis. And, fifth, without explicit management support, the time pressures on, and implicit incentives for, analysts to focus on current production have made the pursuit of curiosity difficult. In contrast, within the scientific community, "investigator-initiated" research is a primary contributor to discovery and innovation, as well as a powerful factor in validating the research of others. The Intelligence Community has need of just such a procedure.

Over the past decade, the Intelligence Community has made several attempts to redirect attention to long-term research and products that reflect such efforts, but, without a sustained base of interested customers in the senior policy community, these have not succeeded.[23] Analysts have seen the emphasis on the President's Daily Brief (PDB) and similar serial products as a clear indication of where interest (and therefore success) is to be found.[24] Although some suggest that current intelligence can provide the basis for deep understanding, it seems obvious that attempting to achieve this by compiling current reporting is not a satisfactory method for producing integrated, synoptic analyses that are set in full context. A better route to meeting the competing demands of producing both current intelligence and deep analytical products would be to exploit the expertise and domain understanding of the experienced analysts doing in-depth research to identify, select, extract, and put into context the important tidbits from the reporting stream—and to use those as a basis for more in-depth and sustained exchanges with users of intelligence.

7. The Neglect of Anticipatory Intelligence

The "information revolution" has unsettled intelligence officials by providing policymakers with alternative sources for both coverage of developments and in-depth research and understanding on issues of interest to them, as well as allowing them to become their own intelligence analysts, if they so choose. These trends have left Intelligence Community managers struggling to emulate the success of television as the provider of real-time news and has prompted the worrisome notion that customers might now see intelligence as less relevant. But the community must go beyond the current interest areas of its customers if it is to perform its primary national function of preventing surprise. In the new and very dynamic geostrategic environment, perhaps the most important element of warning is the anticipatory function against the unexpected—*discovering* new activities that might prove inimical to US national interests and obtaining information about them. Leads to issues of this kind are not likely to come from customer requests; as noted, in science, "investigator-initiated" research is a particularly important driver for discovery and innovation.

Correcting this problem demands that the leadership of the Intelligence Community be prepared to spend real resources on issues that are not immediately "customer-relevant," even when confronted by what seem to be limitless demands to focus on high-priority subjects. Waiting on the policy community to furnish requirements for anticipatory intelligence all but assures that there will be serious warning failures—and the community will shoulder the blame for the policy-makers "surprise." Faced with its concerns about diminishing relevance, the anticipatory role is one the Intelligence Community should grasp. At the same time, the dichotomy between current situational awareness based on a stream of detailed reporting and anticipatory or predictive intelligence is more apparent against a new enemy who relies on "stilettos and stealth" than it was against the Soviet Union, which amassed large stocks of advanced weapons whose visible and patterned development path took well over a decade and then allowed us to collect hard evidence on them by exercising those capabilities extensively. For a community which frequently restates the mantra that it is "an evidence-based" culture, this divergence of reduced collection capabilities against lower signature targets and the increasing demands for anticipatory judgments resting on long inference chains will create an uncomfortable problem in producing these assessments.

8. The Loss of "Keystone Species" and "Intellectual Middleware"

The relatively recent ecological concept of "Keystone Species" denotes organisms that play a central role within an environment, either as a resource or as a control mechanism. Within the Intelligence Community, the most important of these "keystone species" is perhaps the "journeymen" analysts.[25] These experienced analysts (say, those with seven or more years of analytic experience) are the functional equivalent of doctoral students, post-doctoral fellows, and assistant professors in academia and of the house staff (interns and residents) in medical education, both of which are also guild/craft systems. Journeymen perform the bulk of the work of producing products, making incremental improvements in process, teaching the apprentices, and disseminating knowledge and skills as they move to new communities. The journeymen carry institutional memory, transmit knowledge to junior analysts, and inculcate in them such vital professional values as intellectual curiosity, humility, and an ethos of continual learning. In addition, they form the core of a high-trust social network built on longstanding prior contacts that is essential to the diffusion of knowledge within the Intelligence Community and the national security community as a whole.

Recognizing the journeymen's role as a "keystone species" helps to explain the severe disruptions caused by the disproportionate drawdown in their numbers triggered by the budget cutbacks of the early 1990s. To a considerable extent, this cadre, with its deep professional expertise, was sacrificed because of the disinterest of the policy community; nonetheless, the senior management of the Intelligence Community allowed it to happen. Moreover, increasing pressures for "broadening" rotational assignments and "up-orout" promotion policies make it more difficult to retain the remaining cadre of deeply skilled experts as working analysts.

The loss of journeymen also underscores the crucial importance for the analytical profession of soft cultural factors and people-related processes, such as mentoring. Inadvertently, as mentors disappeared, the important socialization and professionalization processes that are essential to train, guide, and acculturate the current flood of apprentice analysts went with them. A further difficulty is that, absent either emphasis on, or demand for, research products, the departure of experienced analysts and the focus on current intelligence and reporting makes it difficult to train and mature newcomers in creating such deep products.

As a consequence, the community also lost the "intellectual middleware"[26] that was a central element of its knowledge base and what one former senior intelligence officer terms its "ecology of expertise."[27] Intellectual middleware is the profound complementary understanding of both domain and process that is gained from long experience. Along with the knowledge base built-up over years, middleware is a necessary link between current intelligence and deep understanding of a domain; it provides the essential capabilities necessary for either considered in-depth judgments or meaningful quick-response products. As a conference participant with extensive analytic experience noted, "Dick Kerr did a study...of all the analysis that was written on Iraq [by the CIA].... He said...it was very good, there was a lot of detail, there was a lot of information, but he came away from all that analysis having no real sense of what Iraq, the country, was all about."[28] Of course, working on research projects contributes to the production of middleware, which, in turn, serves as a resource for all other products and advice; this is something that working on a succession of current and limited studies can never do.

The Intelligence Community once had a fairly standard method for introducing analysts to the process of research, which was to have them draft a new edition of a lengthy product known as a National Intelligence Survey (NIS). Working on a project such as this created in-depth analytic expertise and domain knowledge on a country or area. Above all, the knowledge gained by producing an NIS would enable an analyst to provide policymakers with the essential context for current intelligence, to render informed judgments, and to produce timely answers to important questions. Unfortunately, the importance of the NIS process was not recognized within the community, and the practice was abandoned.

9. Failure to Develop Analytic Tools and Methods for Validation

Most of the tools available to support analysis provide help for specific analytic techniques or intelligence disciplines, such as imagery intelligence (IMINT) and signals intelligence (SIGINT), rather than for all-source analysis. Even so, there are formal methodologies taught and employed within the community for all-source analysis, especially for assessing and marshalling evidence, and there are structured methods that support hypothesis assessment.[29] Consistent with its "craft" culture, the Intelligence Community has used practical experience rather than formal validation methods to assess utility and select these tools. Rob Johnston has observed, however, that there is a large number of tools and methods available to the analytic community, but few are consistently employed—and none has been tested or validated to assure its effectiveness and utility.[30] As one seasoned analyst commented, "... imagine a nuclear powered Navy in which all the Reactor Plant Operating Manuals are written by the current ship's engineer and whenever he got relieved they were all shredded and the new engineer had to write his own."[31] Of course, as has often been noted by students of intelligence, that an agency or community opinion is wrong does not automatically mean that the process followed in reaching that opinion was flawed.[32] Again, quoting Charles Allen,

> We're not very good at evaluating the quality of intelligence analysis independent of the outcome. We're outcome oriented, rather than process oriented.
>
> Conversely, when the policy succeeds and a desirable outcome occurs, we feel satisfied with the conduct of intelligence and generally look no further. The cumulative effect of this process is that it undermines the very essence of intelligence analysis.[33]

Within the diverse domain of intelligence analysis, one would expect that analytic methods and tools would vary significantly, not only depending on the sources of intelligence available and the subject matter, but also on the epistemology of the question at hand—whether the problem is, to use Fritz Ermarth's typology, a secret, a mystery, or an obscurity. "Secret" means the information exists but must be acquired—usually by clandestine collection methods—and interpreted. A "mystery" is a question for which a set of possible outcomes may be known but whose particular outcome can be known only after the fact. An "obscurity" involves questions that are often unrecognized and not seen to be relevant until they are posed explicitly—which requires curiosity, a quality often in short supply. Data to illuminate obscurities are also often available—even if found in nontraditional sources that require imagination to identify, if procedures to filter signal from noise can be developed, and if appropriate inference chains can be constructed from the evidence. For example, Murray Feschbach drew accurate inferences about the internal strength of the Soviet system from totally "outof-domain," low-level, openly-available statistical data on morbidity and mortality published by the Soviets themselves.[34]

> The Intelligence Community often perceives its comparative advantage with decisionmakers in secret information that only it can access and supply.

The Intelligence Community, however, as a function of its history and culture, has constructed a "hierarchy of privilege" for information that still gives the most weight to secret intelligence. Similarly, many users of intelligence information accord greater credence to reports with higher levels of classification. And, of course, the Intelligence Community often perceives its comparative advantage with decisionmakers in secret information that only it can access and supply. At the same time, unfortunately, the more evidence and judgments are restricted in dissemination by compartmentation and distribution limitations, the more likely it is that questionable judgments will pass unchallenged. This is an especially serious problem for HUMINT, which, by its nature, provides only a very narrow perspective on events for which direct confirmation may not be available. Yet timely, authoritative, and credible HUMINT is sometimes—however rarely—the only way to obtain information that can determine strategic direction.

10. The Hindrances of the Security Mindset

The current security mindset is an additional impediment to cooperation among and within intelligence agencies, between intelligence agencies and policy agencies at all levels of government, and between community analysts and outside expertise resident in both non-government and foreign sources. This mindset is extremely risk averse with respect to potential information loss, and it fosters procedures that make it difficult to pull together and share files of relevant information, to bring fresh perspectives to bear, and to exploit the synergies of expert collaboration. This current security paradigm views problem domains as discrete and separable and insists that protection of information (and, therefore, sources and methods) is more important than effective exploitation and cross-fertilization. Two problem areas, in particular, are the traditional barrier between the intelligence and law enforcement functions and between foreign and domestic intelligence. Under the pressure of countering the terrorist threat, however, these distinctions are eroding.

End Notes

1 See, for example, a bill proposed by Rep. Jane Harman, the "Intelligence Transformation Act of 2004" (HR4104): "The goal...should be to enhance the DNI's ability to coordinate and integrate operations, focus the community on priorities, share information better...and so on, but not detract from the support that cabinet secretaries need and expect from their intelligence organization, and not dilute competitive analysis."

2 One excuse for the very heavy cuts in mid- and senior-level analytic cadres in the early 1990s was that it was necessary to weed out those whose expertise was presumed to be passé and, therefore, no longer needed.

3 See Jack Davis, "Improving CIA Analytic Performance: Strategic Warning," and "Improving CIA Analytic Performance: DI Analytic Priorities."

4 Several retired, formerly very senior, CIA officials have made this point about erosion of professional élan—ethos, ethics, and standards—that help keep the analyst from, as General Kent put it, succumbing to the temptations of prostitution or proselytizing (see footnote 43 on page 22). One attribute of a profession, especially a "learned profession," is that members can work without supervision. This is also one of the characteristics that define journeymen in a craft system.

5 Carmen Medina, "What To Do When Traditional Models Fail," *Studies in Intelligence* 46, no. 3 and Russ Travers, "The Coming Intelligence Failure," *Studies in Intelligence* 40, no. 2.

6 See Berkowitz, 3. That each organization develops tradecraft and evolves practices that may not transfer easily if challenged by new functions complicates the community's ability to shift its focus and assets to meet new challenges.

7 Creation of an "information commons" must be done in full awareness of the problems associated with the conundrum of commons, the conflict for resources between individual

interests and the common good. Garrett Hardin, "The Tragedy of the Commons," *Science* 162 (1968): 1243–8.

[8] It is like the saying, "better to be approximately correct than precisely wrong." Josh Kerbel, "Thinking Straight: Cognitive Bias in the US Debate About China," *Studies in Intelligence* 48, no. 3 (2004).

[9] In this regard, several commentators, among them Sabel, Fishbein, and Treverton, have recognized the potential applicability of practices drawn from "High Reliability Organizations" (HROs). Both this issue and "mindfulness" will be addressed in greater depth in Chapter Four.

[10] This thought owes much to comments by Stephen Marrin in a private communication on 1 November 2004.

[11] *Intelligence and Policy: The Evolving Relationship*, Center for the Study of Intelligence, June 2004, 7.

[12] These are not new problems. Defense Secretary Donald Rumsfeld, as chairman of the Commission on Ballistic Missile Threats, highlighted the failure of executive and legislative leadership to establish appropriate priorities while besieging the community with ad hoc taskings. See Side Letter to the Rumsfeld Report, 18 March 1999, 2.

[13] Those needs and the impediments on access to national systems underwrote the very large military programs known as TIARA (Tactical Intelligence and Related Activities). National systems are also known as National Technical Means, the term used to refer to them in arms control agreements.

[14] In *Network Centric Warfare: Developing and Leveraging Information Superiority*, David S. Alberts, John J. Garstka, and Frederick P. Stein define NCW as "an information superiority-enabled concept of operations that generates increased combat power by networking sensors, decisionmakers, and shooters to achieve shared awareness, increased speed of command, higher tempo of operations, greater lethality, increased survivability, and a degree of self-synchronization. In essence, NCW translates information superiority into combat power by effectively linking knowledgeable entities in the battlespace."

[15] Sabel, 52ff.

[16] See Conclusion 4, *SSCI Report*, 22–23.

[17] Private communication from Fritz Ermarth, 23 January 2005.

[18] See the "Curveball Report," cited in the *SSCI Report*, 482 and 492.

[19] See, for example, the *SSCI Report*, 32–33 and 484.

[20] Jack Davis, "Paul Wolfowitz on Intelligence-Policy Relations," *Studies in Intelligence* 39, no. 5 (1996).

[21] See Chapter Four for a more complete discussion

[22] This is also a problem for newspapers, and it explains why newspapers, with their daily production cycle, are different from magazines, which can afford to pay more attention to sustained investigative journalism.

[23] See Douglas MacEachin, "The Tradecraft of Analysis: Challenge and Change in the CIA," *Studies in Intelligence* 46, no. 3 (2002): 23–28. It is also interesting to note that the NIE on Iraqi WMD was requested by the Senate Select Committee on Intelligence and the Senate Armed Services Committee, not by executive branch policymakers.

[24] See Rob Johnston, *Analytic Culture in the U.S. Intelligence Community*. Indeed, in response to these concerns, the Commission on the Intelligence Capabilities of the U.S. Regarding Weapons of Mass Destruction strongly urged that the PDB not become the centerpiece of the DNI's analytic focus.

[25] "Journeyman" is not used in a pejorative sense, but, rather, in the traditional guild meaning of the term. In CIA parlance, these are now called "fully qualified" analysts. Military homologues are Navy chief petty officers ("chiefs") and Marine gunnery sergeants ("gunnies").

[26] This term from the computer science community denotes software that performs intermediary functions (such as translation and data exchange) between heterogeneous systems, enabling them to function in an integrated, interoperable manner. The connotation of middleware is "glue" that enables not just interoperability but, in this context, also cross-fertilization.

[27] This concept of an "ecology of expertise," articulated by Fritz Ermarth, is a powerful tool for thinking about the Intelligence Community's role.

[28] See *Charlottesville Conference Report*, 6 and Kerr, et al.

[29] See, for example, Hughes and Schum, "Evidence Marshalling and Argument Construction."

[30] Johnston, 72.

[31] Private communication from John Bodnar.

[32] Put another way, "There are too many targets and too many ways of attacking them for even the best intelligence agencies to discover all threats in time to prevent them from happening." Kerr, et al.

[33] Allen, 3.

[34] See, *inter alia*, *Russia's Health and Democratic Crises* and *Russia's Demographic and Health Meltdown*. Feschbach is currently a senior scholar at the Woodrow Wilson Center and Research Professor Emeritus at Georgetown University.

Chapter 4

A PROGRAM FOR TRANSFORMING ANALYSIS

The following sections lay out some fundamental guidelines, or pathways, for transforming analysis, provide a set of principles upon which to base a restructured analysis paradigm, and suggest six specific areas for attention.[1] To be effective, however, necessary changes need to be implemented within the system, not just identified.

Even a cursory look at the fate of previous Intelligence Community reform efforts does not lead to expectations of great success in such an endeavor.

For this reason, the path suggested here offers the opportunity to make some early course corrections that can be initiated without formal sanction and with minimal changes to existing structures and authorities.[2] It also offers the possibility of winning support from the professional intelligence cadre, who must be convinced that the measures recommended are both effective and sensible.

If they are not convinced, institutional inertia, if not outright resistance, will impede change.

For example, groups of analysts could take ownership of these areas proposed for action, thereby legitimating the transformation effort as an organic program instead of one imposed from above.[3]

> *The community still has not recognized that the dominant intelligence problems are not penetrating "denied areas," but understanding "denied minds."*

Developing a New Concept for Analysis

Several recent assessments contend that the Intelligence Community's problems are manifestations of fundamental and systematic problems within each agency's internal processes, cultures, and organizational structures.[4] Moreover, these shortcomings do not result from a flawed community architecture or from insufficient directive authorities and budgetary control over the community as a whole—although they may be aggravated by them.

There are two fundamental challenges in rebuilding analysis, with a substantial degree of contradiction and inherent tension between them. The first is to avoid being confidently wrong (as in the NIE on Iraqi WMD) by staying closer to available evidence. The second is to provide judgments on complex and often unfamiliar adversaries and on their likely behavior based on fragmentary and frequently ambiguous information (as in the circumstances leading up to the 9/11 attack).[5] The community has still not made the shift to recognizing that the dominant intelligence problems are not penetrating "denied areas," but rather understanding "denied minds." This shift requires rethinking not only the types of information that analysts need, but also the nature of the information gathering necessary to provide that information. In terms of the latter, intelligence practitioners will need to accept that the appropriate mechanisms will not be limited to remote clandestine collection systems or case officers.

The larger issue of how to allow a classic hierarchical organization to meet the challenges of a more fluid environment and dynamic networked adversaries must be faced squarely, but it is also an effort well beyond the scope of this study. Recognizing that this factor is important, however, the discussion below does focus on directly addressing the sources of analytic failures, including several problems stemming from a hierarchical organization model that has been both badly applied and misapplied.

Principles for a New Paradigm

A new paradigm should start with a set of basic principles to guide the rebuilding process, restore professional standards to the conduct of analysis, and help redress the effects of evolved dysfunctional practices. These principles should be mutually agreed between the leadership of the Intelligence Community and the cadre of professional analysts as the basis for an "analytic compact" that will affect priorities and taskings as well as incentives and rewards for performance. Furthermore, even if users do not fully agree, they also should understand these principles to be the foundation that guides the analytic community in its work. In the long-term, it is clearly in the interest of policymakers to rebuild the community's expertise and knowledge so that intelligence can provide highly contextualized and meaningful judgments, whether on current or future issues.

The primary purpose of analytic effort is "sense-making" and understanding, not producing reports. ...

These principles ought, above all, to convey that "analysis" needs to be construed broadly and not solely in a narrow, "reductionist" context that seeks to "know" by decomposing a phenomenon into its constituent parts and approaching it analytically only on the basis of induction from detailed evidence. Many complex phenomena may be better comprehended by approaches that are based more on synthesis—that is, understanding the larger picture—by focusing on the relationships among the parts and on the emergent behavior produced by such interactions. These principles—which, of course, are not meant to be exhaustive— will recognize, therefore, that:

PHILOSOPHY AND VALUES

- Analysts must have a "duty of curiosity," and the analytic process must encourage and reward a deep and meaningful understanding of the phenomena under investigation;
- Analysts must be responsible for defining knowledge needs and, therefore, collection requirements; to do this effectively, they must understand collection capabilities and be sensitive to their limitations;
- Analysts must be active participants in developing integrated strategies for collection and analysis, seeking information instead of being merely passive recipients;
- The primary purpose of analytic effort is "sensemaking" and understanding, not producing reports; the objective of analysis is to provide information in a meaningful context, not individual factoids;
- The knowledge discovered and the expertise created when an analyst researches a problem is at least as important as "finished intelligence" products that may result;

- Learning is an activity that is valued highly by both analysts and the organization;
- Not all intelligence need be immediately "actionable;" informing decisionmakers and enhancing the quality of the decision process is a critical objective;
- Intuition and creative thinking, including positing hypotheses to be tested, are as important to analysis as evidence-based inductive approaches.

THE OVERALL APPROACH

- There are different analytic problems, and there are diverse approaches and methods for resolving them; in many cases, appropriate and intuitively usable tools may enable their consistent use and enhance the effectiveness of these approaches;
- There should be no assumed "hierarchy of privilege" of sources or analytic methods; a wider range of methodologies needs to be employed routinely and consistently, not seen as exceptional "alternative" techniques;
- Analytic tools are intended to support, not supplant, rigorous and structured cogitation by human analysts;
- There should be better access to, and exploitation of, open-source information as an element of all-source analysis;
- Deductive hypothesis-based methods should be employed more often as a complement to traditional evidence-based inductive approaches;
- There should be more use of formal tests of diagnosticity of evidence, thereby improving the ability to confirm or deny hypotheses;
- Collaboration during the analytical process should be routine, not exceptional, and workloads should be balanced accordingly;
- Review and assessment—including peer review—must be an integral element of the analysis and should not be conducted only after-the-fact;
- There should be greater recognition of the propaedeutic and heuristic roles of writing—as tools of discovery and learning—for the analyst; writing is not just a method of transmitting information to the user;
- Contrarian methods and "Red Teams" should be a routine part of the analytic process;[6]

- As opposed to the incremental approach, in which new evidence is assessed piecemeal for its effect on the course of judgments made, more use should be made of a "stock-take" approach, in which the entire collection of evidence is reviewed holistically;[7]
- "Process watchers," charged with recognizing cognitive impediments and process failures, should become integral parts of analytic teams;[8]
- In addition to reviewing products at hand, analytic managers and senior Intelligence Community overseers should subject the knowledge base and domain expertise to continual appraisal in order to assess whether the scaffolding of evidence and the inferential reasoning is sufficiently strong to bear the weight of the judgments being made and the policy decisions that may rest upon them.[9]

INTERACTION WITH USERS

- There may not be a "right" answer, and there may be limits on "knowability";
- Users are owed an honest assessment of the quality of evidence, uncertainties in judgments, and the "knowability" of the answer; transparency in the logic chain and application of evidence is essential;
- Such assessments can be better conveyed through conversation and dialogue than through static "finished" products;
- Analysts should expect users to "pull threads" and question judgments in open dialogue.

Analysts should expect users to "pull threads" and question judgments in open dialogue.

MANAGEMENT AND OVERSIGHT

- Management's first responsibility should be to remove impediments to analysts' ability to function effectively; the core management function is to ensure the process is being followed and is adapting as necessary to changing needs;

- Commitment by analysts rather than enforced compliance by managers must become the driving force in renewed analytical practices;
- Management must be knowledgeable about the practice of analysis and must provide appropriately focused incentives for those they supervise;
- Managers must encourage self-awareness, questioning of existing procedures, and striving for continuous improvement;
- The organization should create a "learning environment"—not only for domain knowledge, but also for process and methodological expertise;
- The organization must encourage not only "near-miss" analysis and error detection, but also the consistent reporting of anomalies and errors;
- There should be toleration of first errors, but no tolerance for repeating the same mistake; being wrong will happen, but failing to learn should be subject to sanction.

Cautions and Precautions

- Self-awareness of cognitive biases and institutional prejudices, as well as a more self-reflective manner, should be intrinsic elements of an analyst's mindset;
- There is no "revealed truth," and assertion by reference to evidence or previous "finished" intelligence products is not proof;
- "Truth" is not held solely by the Intelligence Community, either here or abroad;
- "Truth" is also not necessarily the first priority of users' questions, but answers by analysts should be;
- Ongoing re-examination and revalidation of previous judgments is very important; unless care is taken to validate and maintain the currency of the library of finished intelligence, "layering" poses significant dangers for the analytic process;
- Keeping an open mind—framing multiple hypotheses and looking at different potential interpretations of "the evidence"—is essential if locking in premature judgments is to be avoided;
- Regardless of the apparent rigor of the process, an analyst must approach analytic issues with "mindfulness" of the potential pitfalls in

evidence and analytic methods that are being applied to a particular problem;[10]
- Tools and methodologies should be tested and evaluated for analytic effectiveness and usability before adoption, and analysts should have an important role in evaluating them;
- Because "mindfulness" only goes so far in detecting one's own biases and cognitive failings, a supervisory function that watches over the conduct of the process is important;[11]
- Differences in culture and governance mechanisms are real—not all human actions are determined by Western notions of rational thought or Enlightenment values—and they affect societal and individual preferences and decision metrics.

Additionally, if at all possible, the first audience for the knowledge gained should be the peer "community of practice" rather than the policy users.[12] Too much focus on "serving the first customer" may have served to shortchange the depth of analysis and the rigor that would be demanded by knowledgeable peers. Moreover, analysis must pay more attention to how the knowledge is conveyed to the users while, at the same time, recognizing that the message should rest on a "sound story." The analytic process must reinstill a sense that the discipline of writing serves to discover the story, not only to convey it, and appropriate incentives to encourage these behaviors must be instituted.

> If at all possible, the first audience for knowledge gained should be the peer "community of practice" rather than the policy users.

Getting Started: Six Fundamentals

This set of principles provides the basis for a systematic campaign to enhance analytic effectiveness in the three interrelated areas of people, process, and technology. The process dimension defines the characteristics and qualities of the enhancements needed in the people and technology areas, and that is the focus of this study. The people dimension must address, in addition to recruitment and training, impediments to good work and work practices, retention, and professional development, as well as appropriate organizational and institutional incentives to overcome them. The technology dimension must be centered around enabling and facilitating both the people and process dimensions, not simply on updating the technical infrastructure to move more data faster.

The corrective measures proposed here address six processes that are indispensable to restoring the Intelligence Community's capability to perform effective intelligence analysis. These proposals emphasize:

1) A reconceptualized set of processes and procedures (including tools, methods, and practices) for analysis;
2) An integrated process for recruiting, training, educating, and professionalizing analysts based on a traditional graduate education model emphasizing close mentoring;
3) A new, more interactive process for communication between users and intelligence analysts throughout the intelligence cycle;
4) A fundamentally revised process for establishing "proof," validating evidence and judgments, and reviewing those judgments;
5) A process for capturing the lessons of experience and advancing organizational learning; and
6) A process for continual collaboration and sharing.

A Revamped Analytic Process

Effective intelligence analysis requires the coupling of deep expertise with innovative approaches and intuition instead of the constraining formalism of "scientism." Although adopting methods of alternative analysis[13] and setting up red teams are a useful start, creating a more coherent structure and a demanding, self-reflective analytic process must also involve more than calls for lateral, out-of-the-box, or non-linear thinking on the part of individual analysts. Real change must alter the very modes of thought that dominate the expectations and practices of today's users, managers, and creators of all-source analysis. Both "sensemaking" and curiosity should be basic elements of this transformed paradigm.[14]

Models already exist for such a new paradigm, as a review of other domains in which failure of work processes can have large potential adverse consequences demonstrates. These domains fall into two distinct categories: 1) where the standardized procedures may not be sufficient to prevent routine but costly failures and 2) where routine procedures are clearly insufficient to face extraordinary conditions. In all of these models, however, the salient features are a high degree of self-awareness, emphasis on early error detection and correction, and the ethos of a "learning organization."

In the first category are organizations, such as those engaged in manufacturing and transaction processing, which specialize in maximizing the effectiveness of routine operations through continuous attention to improvements in the process. For these organizations, even small variances in outcome are a signal that routine procedures need to be adjusted, or significantly altered, in order to correct errors that cumulatively could become worrisome. These organizations have adopted the emphasis of the Quality Movement on consistent, continual self-examination and improvement; perhaps the best known of these is Toyota with its formalized *kaizen* (continuous improvement) system. Other organizations have implemented similar techniques; among these are the "5 Whys Approach," which focuses on recursive questioning to identify the root causes of failure rather than its superficial symptoms, and the Six Sigma Movement, which emphasizes consistency and reductions in process variance.[15]

In the second category, such domains include the nuclear power industry, civil aviation, and aircraft carrier operations. These organizations recognize that routine operations can produce or face conditions that unexpectedly turn extraordinary, with serious, adverse consequences. The paradigm for organizations of this type is the High Reliability Organization (HRO) model.[16] Some commentators would also include hospitals, and especially their high-risk specialty units, as HROs because of the large consequences of error. Built-in practices— formal protocols, structured procedures, and self-awareness measures such as mortality and morbidity (M&M) conferences— are a sign that hospitals recognize the risks of errors.[17]

A common denominator of both categories of organizations is that they "...reliably forestall catastrophic outcomes through 'mindful' attention to ongoing operations."[18] As Fishbein and Treverton note, quoting Karl Weick and Kathleen Sutcliffe, "The unifying trait of HROs is that they exhibit the quality of 'mindfulness,' defined as:

> ...the combination of ongoing scrutiny of existing expectations, continuous refinement and differentiation of expectations based on new experiences, willingness and capability to invent new expectations that make sense of unprecedented events,...and identification of new dimensions of context that improve foresight and current functioning.[19]

These organizations address the possibility of extraordinary events by building procedures that are designed to do more than maximize effectiveness and efficiency in the conduct of routine operations. The organization is focused on addressing non-routine operations, so that the unexpected "...doesn't surprise or disable them" and "...coping actions seldom make the situation worse."[20] These organizations see small errors in routine operations, in addition to their role as process signals, as indications that organizational compliance and managerial oversight are slipping—and that such slippage could presage worse failures.

> Successful day-to-day operations can give rise to mindlessness, defined as inattention to the environment and to internal procedures. Mindfulness, on the other hand, emphasizes continuous updating and assessing of alternate interpretations and implications of incoming information.

Both categories of organization understand that successful day-to-day operations can give rise, in effect, to *mindlessness*, defined as inattention to the environment and to internal procedures. In these circumstances, people slip into routines, fail to notice changes in a larger context, see new phenomena in old categories, and use incoming information (even if it indicates significant variances) to confirm expectations. *Mindfulness*, on the other hand, emphasizes continuous updating and assessing alternate interpretations and implications of incoming information; even small signs of failure can suggest serious problems in organizational processes and compliance with them. In these organizations, according to Wieck and Sutcliffe, there is a "preoccupation with failure, both past and present"; and there is a concomitant stress on early error detection and correction at the lowest levels, as well as emphasis on error reporting upwards as part of the self-assessment "contract."[21]

> The process watcher function is intended to focus exclusively on identifying errors in the analytic process, not on alternative interpretations of the evidence or different logic chains.

Each category contains proven features that recommend themselves for inclusion in a new synthesis for a transformed intelligence analysis process.[22] ***From the High Reliability Organization***, the feature is "mindfulness," which is composed of five processes (and sub-processes below them): anticipating and becoming aware of the unexpected; containing the unexpected; near-miss analysis; active management; and enhancing containment. The most important elements in creating an anticipatory capability are a reluctance to simplify interpretations, which increases blind spots by filtering and abstracting key details; recognizing the effect of categorization on expectations by continually reexamining categories and event coding; and reassessing the basic assumptions and keystones of one's analysis and analysis process. In addition, the stress on "near-miss analysis" is designed to recognize imperfections and errors before they cause consequential failures.

> Both [near-miss and line stoppages in a just-in-time system] trigger root-cause analysis meant to uncover not only the proximate cause of the incident, but to eliminate, through redesign of the organization if necessary, the background conditions which generated the immediate source of the danger.[23]

From the Quality Movement, the synthesis model adopts the "5 Whys Approach," employing a recursive questioning process that emphasizes the importance of identifying root causes of errors. This involves looking beyond the obvious first answer to the "what went wrong" question to the serially deeper causes until the base source of error is found. From medicine, there are two elements worth including. First is the practice of mortality and morbidity conferences, which focus on both near-miss and failure analysis. The second is the practice of "grand rounds" in which house staff, students, and attending physicians brief and review especially difficult cases. Both measures underscore the importance of open and collaborative communication in identifying and assessing hard problems, including both those that were resolved successfully and those that failed. Such open communication is essential to both investigatory and teaching roles. Finally, the introduction of a "process watcher," as suggested by Kahneman, is intended to bring a clear and unbiased, outside expert's eye to analytic teams. The process watcher function, unlike that of a Red Team, is intended to focus exclusively on identifying errors in the analytic process, not on alternative interpretations of the evidence or different logic chains.

In light of the real challenges to conducting complex analysis effectively, it is important that the Intelligence Community identify and evaluate tools and methodologies that can help analysts make sense of complex phenomena rife with ambiguous or incomplete evidence—and then actually provide them. The revamped paradigm must also include processes that are more specifically directed toward strengthening the practice and content of analytic methods. This paradigm would very likely incorporate more widespread and routinized use of formalized techniques, such as Analysis of Competing Hypotheses

(ACH), to explore multiple hypotheses and would employ appropriate supporting tools to facilitate their use.[24] There would also be more emphasis on the use of negative evidence and on its implications for key assumptions and inferences, especially when the orientation is toward current intelligence.[25] Finally, new collaborative mechanisms, such as "blogs" (web logs), "wikis" (wikipedia entries), and groupware could be employed to facilitate better communication and a more continuous dialogue among the parties within the community of interest.[26]

This new analytic paradigm is designed to lead analysts to reflect more intensively on the practice of their trade. It is also intended to develop more structured procedures and to instill in both individual analysts and analytic units the discipline to follow them. Such changes will need to be implemented carefully, so as not to interfere with individual creative processes and existing analytic practices that are effective, especially those that are unorthodox and not easy to assess with formalized metrics. It will be especially important to guard against the danger that too much introspection will cause analysts to avoid risk by dodging judgments.

RECRUITING, TRAINING, EDUCATING, AND DEVELOPING PROFESSIONALS

In the wake of 9/11, the Intelligence Community has been able to take advantage of an upwelling of public support to tap a large pool of candidate analysts. These candidates are, on the surface, talented, diverse, and well educated; but they will require extensive training and professionalization in order to become effective and productive contributors to the analytic community. Furthermore, in current circumstances, when analysts should more frequently be addressing the challenge of "discovery" and open-ended, undefined problems than more readily defined monitoring tasks, they are confronted by time pressures that leave them with little latitude for reflection and wondering. Moreover, our educational system increasingly produces linear thinkers more comfortable "painting within the lines" and pointed more toward likely solutions than toward broader problem-solving capabilities.[27] It is unclear if these shortcomings can be corrected by better-targeted recruitment and more effective training, or if it must be addressed by redesigning fundamental processes and practices; it is likely that both tracks will be needed.

However the question of academic preparation is resolved, rebuilding the apprenticeship and mentoring system is crucial. It is essential, therefore, to reconstitute the "keystone species" represented by the journeyman analyst.[28] This cannot be done by bringing in a flood of young, inexperienced analysts; dousing them with a short period of classroom training (begrudged by their managers and mostly focused on the right tone and format for reports); and leaving them to learn good practices while sifting for nuggets of current intelligence.

There is no known mechanism that can turn the apprentices into "instant" journeymen; they cannot be transformed by lectures, abstract study, or classroom exercises; nor can software tools enable them to substitute for more experienced analysts.[29] This challenging task demands a focused, directed effort at deep analysis within a subject area, most likely through a tutoring and apprenticeship model.[30] In addition, revised classroom instruction, based on a significantly strengthened curriculum emphasizing analytic methodologies and methods, could have an important role within a rebuilt program for professional development. The Intelligence Community should move away from "training courses" that take analysts off-line for weeks to months and reintegrate this type of training directly into the "practice" of intelligence analysis, as is done in clinical education for medicine and law. Moreover, it is absolutely essential to create a professional "duty of curiosity," which the training process would embed in the professional ethos and management would encourage, even in the face of time pressures to meet priority taskings. Further, a peripatetic career for senior analysts— "moving around to move up," often increasingly farther from the actual practice of analysis—is not a useful way to foster deep expertise or to create effective role models. Reestablishing a new cadre of effective professional intelligence analysts will require basic changes in their career patterns, potentially requiring that the military practice of tracking and protecting vital sub-specialties with their own career ladders be emulated.

As an Intelligence Analyst's Rite of Passage Might Look

As the Stefiks made admirably clear in their book about innovation:

Graduate school is a rite of passage for becoming researchers and inventors. Graduate schools create the next generation of researchers and inventors who are primed to step into positions in the world of science and innovation.

> The experience of graduate school draws on a much earlier tradition than undergraduate education, or even high school and grammar school. Education prior to graduate school is dominated by a program of lectures, exercises and exams.
>
> Such educational practices have a predetermined curriculum intended to serve classes of students essentially in lock step....
>
> In contrast, graduate school is based on the older tradition of mentoring and apprenticeship. Graduate education is about assisting students to take on a professional practice. The curriculum is more tailored. Students acquire the practice by working with multiple mentors, adjusting the emphasis to fit their career objectives. Students discover, sometimes by osmosis, elements of practice that would seldom be encountered in a classroom setting. Graduation requires demonstrated mastery at the level of a practitioner in the field.[1]
>
> [1] Stefik and Stefik, 85.

These factors prompt the thrust to restructure the career path of intelligence analysts, perhaps along the lines of medical or science graduate education—especially doctoral and post-doctoral—that integrates classroom learning, research, and clinical practice. In neither case are education and training separated; each is seen as an integral element in producing a practicing member of the medical or scientific community. In this context, then, deeper analytical products are essential to building the process expertise and domain knowledge of the analyst and to rebuilding the domain knowledge base. Together, these capabilities enable a skilled analyst to contextualize current intelligence for the decisionmaker.

Such a restructured program should also seek to foster an open seminar atmosphere during the training process and impart to analysts the practice of critical collaborative discussion within a professional network carried directly into the workplace. Moreover, in this process, in which socialization is seen as an important aspect of absorbing the ethics and ethos that should guide a professional, a close relationship with a mentor is crucial. The mentorship process also reinforces the HRO's emphasis on a "culture of learning," a habit of error reporting developed by encouraging openness, tolerance of even "stupid questions," and professional collaboration as a norm.

The drastic shortages in the cadre of experienced analysts prompt three final thoughts on this process. First, the Intelligence Community must bring back sufficient mentors (even if on contracts that permit double-dipping), so that it can truly support the apprenticeship model with highly personalized mentoring. This will not be an easy task; mentors will need to be chosen carefully and supervised properly, so that the right lessons from experience are passed on— not cynical views carried away from previous experience with a dysfunctional process. Second, the community also needs to give up the conceit that it can develop software and tools that will make the novices into journeymen or experts without their going through this lengthy process of apprenticeship. This is not to say, however, that appropriate tools either do not exist or cannnot be developed to help them do their jobs better and perhaps progress through the cycle more quickly. Third, and perhaps most important in the interim, the Intelligence Community should look for alternative ways to produce the intelligence insights that the journeymen used to provide while, at the same time, reestablishing the vital interrelated processes that created and fostered the development of "intellectual middleware." During this effort, managers must avoid the temptation to use these mentors to supplement the analytic cadre or to force the apprentices to rush their "analytical" fences.

About Apprenticeships

There is often a gap between what can be learned in formal lessons and what needs to be conveyed in total....

When graduate students begin working with their mentors, they are embarking on a journey with an experienced guide. Apprenticeship amounts to going around the research cycle a few times, asking questions, and getting help at the trickier steps.[1]

[1] Stefik and Stefik, 86.

USER-COMMUNITY INTERACTIONS

The current processes for interaction between the Intelligence Community and its consumers, especially senior policymakers, do not work well at either end of the "Intelligence Cycle." The community does a less than satisfactory job of communicating its judgments to these customers.[31] At the same time, few users have any real education or understanding of the Intelligence Community's capabilities and limitations. To a large degree, both problems can be ascribed to too little sustained dialogue, interaction, engagement, or mutual understanding; both parties fail to understand that they are in a collective process of discovery, sensemaking, and judgment. These failings have not come about by accident, however, but by community preference. They flow from what have been deeply rooted beliefs—especially strong at CIA—that too close an association with policymakers and their political concerns runs the danger of contaminating "pristine" intelligence analyses with "policy judgments."[32] As noted earlier, maintaining an appropriate degree of objectivity is a difficult problem; but a good solution is to be found neither by substituting users' judgments for those of intelligence professionals nor by the professionals ignoring users' real interests and needs.

Since the collapse of the Soviet Union, this mutual lack of understanding, combined with the lack of a sustained strategic policy that would provide consistent guidance and priorities, has forced the Intelligence Community to divine targets and priorities from immediate customer requirements rather than from a longer time horizon with a more strategic, synoptic, and open-minded field of view. Moreover, this tendency was reinforced throughout most of the 1990s by budget pressures that drove the community to focus on issues "relevant" to senior policy-makers —and, therefore, defensible in budget hearings. Unfortunately, this approach guarantees myopia, and the Intelligence Community winds up bearing the blame for "failures" to see threats from outside the policymakers' fields-of-vision.

> Analysts and their managers should be prepared to be forthright in admitting what they don't know and in identifying explicitly the uncertainties in judgments they provide.

The current "over-the-transom" process for taskings and questions often leaves the working analyst without a good understanding of the real issues at stake or the purposes to which customers will put the answers once delivered. Yet, both are important if uncertainties and sources are to be addressed in a context that the policy-maker can appreciate. When the Intelligence Community provides its analyses and judgments, too much emphasis is given to the format in which the information is presented, and there is too little real dialogue with the users. The layout—too frequently formal, precisely-formatted, sterile "finished products"—often masks uncertainties and points of contention unless the reader is witting enough to "pull the threads," an effort that can lead to charges of politicization.

The community should move away from the notion that "finished intelligence" conveys certainty; highlighting and clarifying disagreements, especially over fundamental assumptions and judgments, would be of more value to high-level policymakers.[33] At the same time, the false expectations conveyed by the "conceit of finished intelligence" and the "illusion of omniscience" must be changed on both sides. Users must learn that there may not be a "right" answer; that the "more probable" case in the forecast set may not be the situation that will eventuate; and that, therefore, a range of thoughtful (and thought through) contingency responses may be necessary.

Equally, analysts and their managers should be prepared to be forthright in admitting what they don't know and in identifying explicitly the uncertainties in judgments they provide. This means providing greater transparency and traceability as they construct inference chains based on explicitly denoted qualified evidence, other information, assumptions, and hypotheses.[34] Analysts must themselves remember and remind policymakers of Heisenberg's rule: that we are not simply outside observers of a process who have no effect on the outcome; our perceptions and actions are integral elements in a multiplayer game with strongly coupled feedback loops and action-reaction cycles.[35] Finally, it must be recognized that the frequent lack of deep understanding of intelligence on the part of its primary policy users suggests that a serious education effort needs to be undertaken.

Members of other communities—the strategic nuclear community may be the best example—deal with arcane subjects that must be communicated clearly to national decisionmakers who often lack experience or expertise in such matters. They have addressed this problem by developing formal procedures for educating their users and managing their expectations.

Unfortunately, if all the policymakers see is a continuous flow of "current information" while lacking deep knowledge of a topic or the time to synthesize and integrate what they do learn into a coherent picture, an Intelligence Community version of Gresham's law may well apply—factoids devoid of context will drive out thinking. This situation has implications not only for management of the technical systems that support and encourage collaboration and sharing, but also for the important social aspects of group behavior and the mechanisms for interaction between policy users and the analysts. It has significant implications both for the roles intelligence analysts will play and for the modalities through which they produce and communicate their analyses to users.

> The community needs to create processes that capture the best of the legal system's adversarial model and the scientific community's horizontal peer review.

Communicating complex judgments and degrees of confidence in those judgments is best done through conversation among the parties, which demands different mechanisms than simple dissemination of "facts." If the mechanisms for interaction with the users of intelligence are designed only to support the provision of individual pieces of evidence rather than to engage both parties in an extended conversation in which ambiguity and subtlety can be communicated, it is unlikely that either party will be satisfied with these interactions. Indeed, it is worth asking whether the Intelligence Community has any unique contributions to make to anticipatory judgments compared with what policymakers can provide themselves, and, if so, what are they? Posing the question this way emphasizes that such anticipatory assessments are in the realm of judgment, an area that the community, in its quest for "rigor," has often tried to avoid. Now, given the variety of alternative information sources available to the policymaker, is even superb "current reporting" enough to make the community essential, especially to the policy users?

"Proof," Validation, and Review

Failures in the pre-war estimates concerning Iraq's WMD capabilities highlight deep-seated problems in the extremely "self-referential"—that is, customarily internal, collegial, and lacking rigor—process for reviewing and validating intelligence judgments. At the same time, there is absolutely no excuse for allowing easily correctable errors, such as "Key Judgments" that differ from the body of the text or references to earlier assessments that portray their judgments inaccurately, to be conveyed to consumers.[36] The existing process relies fundamentally on an analyst-level coordination process augmented by a hierarchical review process, most often by managers who possess less specific knowledge and are farther removed from the craft of analysis. The community needs to create new processes that capture the best of the legal system's adversarial model of open combat and the scientific community's truly horizontal peer review and independent replication, sprinkling in alternative analyses and red teams to do so on both process and substance.

> To understand "what works" and "what doesn't work," the Intelligence Community should establish an institutional "lessons- learned" process.

Such processes, even if conducted totally inside the community, are bound to be distressing, as knowledgeable individuals subject an analyst's evidence, assumptions, hypotheses, and logic to increased scrutiny. These mechanisms, including workshops and roundtables, would be useful; but if they are composed solely of Intelligence Community members, or those who defer to them, then the problem of a self-referential "proof process" will continue. Therefore, painful as it might prove to be, the Intelligence Community must step outside its usual circle and exploit a wider range of expertise.

In addition to peer review, the scientific community has fostered a range of self-correcting features, such as tension between experimentalists and theoreticians. It also relies on a wider range of alternative proof models. Such additional mechanisms for validation should be examined for incorporation in the revamped intelligence analysis process. Furthermore, as in medicine, law, and science, mechanisms need to be developed and implemented to ensure that knowledge bases are updated and corrected as necessary and that users are notified of major errors in previous reports, so that the cumulative knowledge base is as accurate as possible.[37]

Finally, both the Intelligence Community and its users must have an accurate calibration of whether intelligence is "on top" of important issues and domains. The review process must go beyond assessments of individual products and personnel performance to create processes that assess the "state of knowledge" and the community's (and its users') awareness of that state. This type of self-diagnosis is badly needed, especially as it creates an environment for self-criticism combined with a license to look at the adequacy of information both on specific issues and across wide domain areas.

Key Questions in Reviewing Lessons Learned

Veteran analyst Charles Allen provides a list of questions that a lessons-learned process can assist in answering:

- What set of hypotheses was being considered? Was the set comprehensive, or was there bias in the selection of hypotheses? What *a priori* probability was attached to each hypothesis? Again, was there bias?
- Was there a good understanding about the observables that were expected to differentiate between the hypotheses? Was intelligence collection requested on the basis of these differentially diagnostic observables?

- Were all the available data considered? How were the data weighted? What degree of credibility was accorded the sources?
- Was the possibility of deception considered and accounted for?
- Was the analytic process logically correct? Was the confidence in rendered judgments correctly estimated? If so, and if the confidence was low, was additional collection requested?
- Were the judgments presented in a timely and adequate manner?
- And, of course, was intelligence collection responsive and timely?[1]

[1] Allen, 3–4

After-Action Reports and Lessons-Learned Processes

Unlike medicine or law, militaries do not usually have the luxury of a continuous stream of real opportunities to "practice" their craft or profession. To address these problems, the US military counts on intensive individual and unit training, institutionalized after-action reports and lessons- learned processes, and the exercise of complete operational organizations before units participate in actual operations. It also instantiates understanding of what works best as formal "doctrine" that can be studied and inculcated to provide a common frame of reference and instinctive procedural basis. One can find very similar systems created in both academia and medicine to educate and train their incoming members. In these other professions, there is little distinction or separation between education, research, and training; rather, there is a continuum of learning that depends heavily on the "hands-on" transmission of domain knowledge and process expertise.

In order to understand both "what works" and "what doesn't work," the Intelligence Community should establish an institutionalized lessons-learned process. This would include not only postmortems on major failures but also on successes and near misses.[38]

The purpose of this process is not to assign blame, which is traditionally an inspector general function, nor is it to punish; rather, it should serve as an aid to individual and organizational learning. Both after action reports, developed originally at the US Army's National Training Center (NTC), and lessons-learned processes, used by the Army and the US Joint Forces Command (JFCOM), are effective methods and would be good starting points for creating an Intelligence Community effort.

A good complement to the lessons-learned process is the use of wargaming and scenario methods, developed on an accurate historical basis, to force the participants to examine the situation, the players, their interactions, and the outcomes in a thoughtful manner.

After action reports and lessons-learned processes can also furnish objective evidence of the utility of tools and methodologies and their suitability for addressing various kinds of problems. Without such a measured baseline of effective procedures, methods, and tools, it is difficult to create consistent processes to select and adopt appropriate analytic methodologies or to train and exercise personnel.

In addition, a baseline makes credit assignment and personnel efficiency reviews more reliable. As another former analyst and thoughtful observer of the analytic process has written,

> The identification of causes of past failure leads to kernels of wisdom in the form of process modifications that could make the intelligence product more useful. A more effective, more accurate intelligence capability may still be vulnerable to the cognitive and institutional pathologies that cause failure, but a self-conscious and rigorous program based on the lessons derived from the existing literature would strengthen the intelligence product.[39]

Collaboration

Several of the recent investigations point to the important role in these intelligence failures of lapses in sharing information and coordinating efforts among the constituent elements of the Intelligence Community. Not surprisingly, the suggested remedies often involve establishing new directive authorities to mandate coordination and collaboration and build or improve the technical information infrastructures that could support collaborative activities. In fact, solutions do not start with either directive authorities or new IT systems, although an improved, technically sophisticated information infrastructure would help.

Rather, effective collaboration is fundamentally a matter of culture and values; what is needed is, first, to create appropriate incentive structures for sharing and, second, to forge expert social networks and effective "distributed trust" systems. These are problems of organizational culture that demand active leadership at all levels of management throughout the community.

> Sharing of private information among experts is task for which technical solutions exist, but the community's technical, organizational, cultural, and incentive structures fail to support it.

Moreover, as mentioned previously, the success of the Intelligence Community depends on the promotion of an entire set of effective collaborations: among analysts; between analysts and collectors; between analysts and operations officers; between analysts and the intelligence users; and not least, between community analysts and information sources outside the intelligence or national security enterprise. For example, tasks such as target assessment and collection planning involve complex collaborative activity among analysts and collectors. Often there are subtle bits of information that appear significant only in the context of tidbits from other disciplines or aspects of tradecraft which may be little understood— or not at all—outside the ranks of its own practitioners. Each of these collaborations involves a distinct "community of interest" or "community of practice" and represents a different type of social construct; none is fundamentally dependent on building more elaborate technical infrastructures as its primary need. Fostering effective collaborations can serve an important bootstrapping function as well, because participants in the collaboration are likely to become effective champions of more collaboration.

Furthermore, true collaboration within the Intelligence Community should address more than simply sharing raw intelligence among different analytic components or taking part in the coordination process for finished products. The Intelligence Community understands how to do these tasks, even if they are not implemented effectively today. The real challenge and greatest leverage will come from sharing private information, initial hypotheses and tacit knowledge, among networks of experts in order to increase the opportunities for discovery of previously unrecognized significance. This is a task for which technical solutions are now known and feasible, but the community's technical, organizational, cultural, and incentive structures fail to support it. A true collaborative environment must build effective trust systems among community analysts and collectors, especially between the DI and the DO. Indeed, such trusted environments should extend beyond the Intelligence Community to policymakers and, eventually, to other sources of expertise outside of the community and even outside the United States.

Another important reason for fostering collaboration is that of reducing information costs. Such reductions can result not only from the powerful impacts of information technologies on organizational forms, but also from the role of "social networks" as a medium for sharing among trusted members. Such networks, especially those among journeymen analysts, substantially reduce the transaction costs of creating and transmitting knowledge; in particular, they are a low-cost information resource for the essential tacit knowledge, both domain and process, that is so difficult to elicit and instantiate in formal knowledge systems.

Moreover, because of the wide-ranging social network that journeymen build over their years of service, these networks can both help to diffuse account-specific insights into other areas and infuse other perspectives into their domain, often cutting across formal community security compartmentation restrictions. As with many examples of military C2, it is these informal networks and processes that truly enable the system to function. The potential of using "groupware," such as Groove and other collaboration platforms, in building and strengthening these social networks bears careful exploration and experimentation.[40]

Finally, the Intelligence Community's security mindset should also be addressed. The overall approach to security—mandated from the top by the newly created DNI if it is to have sufficient weight to become the new paradigm—must move away from the existing risk-averse model, which really seeks to avoid problems.

Despite the likelihood of significant opportunity costs, the direction must be toward a risk management model like that increasingly being adopted for information security in other government agencies and the private sector. One approach would take responsibility for personnel and IT security out of the hands of dozens of individual agencies and make them the responsibility of a single community manager who would also have the power to adjudicate equities and make risk management decisions.[41]

A single authority under the new DNI would issue security clearances and set security requirements for IT that would apply throughout the federal government (or at least the executive branch), among government contractors, and, ideally, to state and local government agencies, as required. This system would also eliminate the need to have clearances passed, making expedient collaboration easier.

Uniform security standards for IT systems could make the electronic sharing of information and on-line collaboration among analysts substantially easier, thereby enabling the formation of collaborative "communities of interest" within a secure information environment.

End Notes

[1] A comprehensive discussion of remedial measures is beyond the scope of this paper.

[2] Several reviewers, all of whom are experts in management theory and organizational behavior, suggested this idea in parallel.

[3] See Michael Mears, "The Intelligence Community Genome: RIA Paper #3." It is an insightful look at the practical challenges of organizational transformation in the Intelligence Community.

[4] See Jeffrey Cooper, "Intelligence & Warning: Analytic Pathologies," and Johnston.

[5] See Kerr, et al. for a more extensive discussion by seasoned analysts on improvements needed in analysis.

[6] Composition of the teams, however, might better be rotational and *ad hoc*. See also Kerr, et al., 52: "Indeed, although certain gaps were acknowledged, no product or thread within the intelligence provided called into question the quality of basic assumptions...."

[7] The "stock-take" originated in the UK atomic weapons program; it differs fundamentally from the more usual practice, which holds that new information will appropriately correct earlier judgments. But this approach, based on Bayesian logic, depends on the earlier "priors," which may never be carefully reexamined.

[8] Professor Daniel Kahneman, who teaches at Princeton University, also suggested this approach in the slightly different military "command and control" (C2) context in an interview with me in October 2000. Johnston discusses this approach at length in his chapter on "Integrating Methodologists into Teams of Experts."

[9] Fritz Ermarth made this suggestion in a communication to me on 23 January 2005.

[10] See Warren Fishbein and Gregory Treverton, *Rethinking "Alternatives Analysis" to Address Transnational Threats.*

[11] The standard approach to addressing bias and prejudice in judgment and decisionmaking has been through training to recognize one's own cognitive errors. During my research on cognitive impediments to C2 decisionmaking for the Defense Advanced Research Projects Agency (DARPA), Professor Daniel Kahneman pointed out that this approach has not succeeded, despite more than 25 years of trying. Kahneman was awarded the Nobel Prize in Economics for his work on imperfections in decisionmaking. (Personal interview, October 2000.)

[12] This issue was highlighted in Rozak, *et al.*

[13] See Fishbein and Treverton, 2, for a succinct and useful discussion of "alternatives analysis."

[14] "Sensemaking" in this context means the ability to perceive, analyze, represent, visualize and make sense of one's environment and situation in a contextually appropriate manner. See both Fishbein and Treverton, 3, and Cooper, "*Sensemaking: Focusing on the Last Six Inches*."

[15] See the Six Sigma website, http://www.isixsigma.com/.

[16] A number of perceptive commentators have pointed to HRO as a useful model, although often for diverse reasons. See Sabel, Johnston, and Stephen Marrin in "Preventing Intelligence Failures by Learning from the Past," and Fishbein and Treverton.

[17] The continuing high rates of medical errors and the increasing appearance of "iatrogenic" (that is, physician-induced) diseases in hospitals suggest, however, that these organizations have a long way to go before they can be fully recognized as HROs.

[18] Karl E. Weick and Kathleen M. Sutcliffe, *Managing the Unexpected: Assuring High Performance in an Age of Uncertainty*, 23.

[19] Fishbein and Treverton, 4, quoting Weick and Sutcliffe, 25.

[20] Weick and Sutcliffe, 42.

[21] Weick and Sutcliffe, quoted in Fishbein and Treverton.

[22] This study will develop a brief outline of such organizational characteristics, but a comprehensive treatment will require a separate paper.

[23] Sabel, 30.

[24] An example is the ACH Tool developed by Palo Alto Research Center (PARC) for the Novel Intelligence from Massive Data (NIMD) Program under the Intelligence Community's Advanced Research and Development Activity (ARDA).

[25] Kerr, et al.

[26] See Calvin Andrus's Galileo Award winning paper, "Toward a Complex Adaptive Intelligence Community," in *Studies in Intelligence* 49, no. 3 (2005).

[27] As Daniel Goleman noted in his answer to the "2005 *Edge* Question," an annual survey by *The Edge*, an internet site favored by the technical community.

[28] Additional incentives to retain these experts appear worth considering.

[29] Frank J. Hughes, *Preparing for the Future of Intelligence Analysis.*

[30] Hughes, 2–3

[31] The term "Intelligence Cycle" is itself part of the problem. With its Industrial Age antecedents, it usually conveys the notion of a self-contained "batch" process rather than a continuous spiral of interactions.

[32] See Davis, "Kent-Kendall Debate."

[33] See Kerr, et al. on "Integration with the Policy Community," 52.

[34] This has important and challenging implications for the estimative methods used by a community self-defined as "evidence-based."

[35] German mathematician Werner Heisenberg (1901-1976). I am indebted to John Bodnar for highlighting this issue.

[36] See *SSCI Report*, 286 and 300.

[37] This problem is significantly aggravated by the lack of a coherent information infrastructure.

[38] This is very much like Klein's "premortems," cited in Fishbein and Treverton, 7. See also Gary Klein, *Intuition at Work: Why Developing Your Gut Instinct Will Make You Better at What You Do*, 88.

[39] Stephen Marrin, "Preventing Intelligence Failures by Learning from the Past," *International Journal of Intelligence and Counterintelligence*, 2004. A recent conference on lessons learned, sponsored by the Center for the Study of Intelligence, discussed this question at some length and provides an excellent point-of-departure for implementation projects. See *Intelligence Lessons Learned Conference*.

[40] Groove is a software package that creates a virtual private network (VPN) within an information network that controls access to a shared collaborative space and provides a variety of tools to facilitate information sharing and collaboration. It is accepted by some components of the Intelligence Community as secure and trustworthy, but it is not widely employed at this time.

[41] The IRTPA, creating the Information Sharing Executive Program Manager, does mandate this, at least for counterterrorism information.

APPENDIX: THE ANALYTIC PATHOLOGIES METHODOLOGY

The "Analytic Pathologies" methodology expands the typical portrayal of the five-part intelligence cycle (planning and direction, collection, processing, analysis and production, and dissemination) to include seven elements in the analytic process:

- question specification and subject understanding
- evidence acquisition and situation perception/assessment
- problem/hypothesis specification
- decision metrics and procedures
- analysis, assessment, and answer preparation
- communication with the client
- feedback and post-hoc assessment.

More consistent with current research on judgment and decisionmaking, this expansion permits a closer look at the analytic process itself. This approach also makes it possible to capture explicitly the important calibration functions of interactions with clients in framing questions and in delivering answers, and it highlights the importance of explicit feedback for self-assessment. In this approach it is also possible to identify more completely the impediments to analysis and to specify the location and distorting effects of each step in the process.

Finally, the methodology explicitly lays out the key processes and functions (as well as impediments) at three organizational levels: individual analysts, work groups and agencies, and the Intelligence Community as a whole. This layout enables investigators to examine the causes of analytic problems and locate their organizational sources; these problems can occur not only where they directly interfere with the analytic process, but also in the functions which support agency and community analytical processes. With that information, appropriate corrective measures can be identified more easily.

Thus, although the Intelligence Community organizational level provides direction, priorities, and controls budgetary resources— which are important support mechanisms and enablers of output functions—it does not itself directly perform any intelligence functions, except analyses conducted by the National Intelligence Council (NIC), now a part of the office of the Director of National Intelligence.

IC Functions and Outputs at Three Levels

Level	Key Functions	Outputs
Intelligence Community	• Direction and Leadership • Setting Priorities • Budgetary Control	• Policies • Oversight • Budgetary Allocation
Work Group/Agency	• Training and Acculturation • Work Practices and Habits (TTPs) • Rewards and Incentives • Review Processes • Organizational Knowledge Base	• Review • Production • Dissemination • Customer Interfaces • Work Processes • Technical Infrastructure • Organizational Culture
Individual	• Analytic Expertise • Domain Knowledge	• Answers • Hypotheses • Knowledge Products • Increased Knowledge • On-demand Expertise

The effectiveness of the Analytic Pathologies methodology as a diagnostic tool suggests its potential utility when used as a framework for developing corrective measures. The diagnostic effort highlights the importance of properly identifying the organizational level at which impediments impinge upon successful analytic practice, as well as the level at which corrective actions must be taken to restore important functions—and these are often not the same. For example, there are a substantial number of impediments to effective performance by individual analysts, but the appropriate corrective measures need to be instituted at the group or organizational level instead of the analytical level. Different corrective measures also have different time constants of effectiveness to be accommodated, both in planning and in measuring improvement; otherwise, phasing conflicts could easily induce resonant oscillation in processes and control mechanisms.

The explicit differentiation among these elements allowed by this methodology can enable individual and organizations at all levels to develop tools to recognize and use pathology self-assessments. It also allows the development of appropriate measures of effectiveness or indicators of performance targeted at relevant outputs rather than inputs. Thus, extending the Analytic Pathologies framework to use as the basis for developing corrective measures offers promise that it may be able to identify and, therefore, avoid perverse consequences that might result from altering structures and processes while attempting to make them more effective.

Bibliography

Alberts, David S, John J. Garstka, Frederick P. Stein. *Network Centric Warfare: Developing and Leveraging Information Superiority.* Washington DC: C4ISR Cooperative Research Program, 1999.

Allen, Charles. "Comments of the Associate Director of Central Intelligence" for Collection at a Public Seminar on Intelligence at Harvard University, spring 2000. (<http:// pirp.Harvard.edu/pdf-blurb.asp?id+518>.)

Andrus, Calvin, "Toward a Complex Adaptive Intelligence Community: The Wiki and the Blog." *Studies in Intelligence* 49, no. 3 (2005).

Armstrong, Fulton. "Ways to Make Analysis Relevant but Not Prescriptive." *Studies in Intelligence* 46, no. 3 (2002).

Barger, Deborah. "It Is Time to Transform, Not Reform, US Intelligence," *SAIS Review of International Affairs* 24, no. 1 (Winter-Spring 2004).

Berkowitz, Bruce. "Intelligence for the Homeland." *SAIS Review of International Affairs* 24, no. 1 (Winter-Spring 2004).

Bodnar, John. *Warning Analysis for the Information Age: Rethinking the Intelligence Process*. Washington, DC: Joint Military Intelligence College, July 2004.

Black, Cofer. "Testimony by Ambassador Cofer Black, Coordinator for Counterterrorism, Before the House International Relations Committee '9/11 Commission Report Recommendations,'" Washington, DC, 19 August 2004. http/wwwc.house.gov/internationalrelations/108/bla 081 904.htm.

Center for the Study of Intelligence. *Intelligence and Policy: The Evolving Relationship*. Washington, DC: Central Intelligence Agency, Center for the Study of Intelligence, June 2004.

Center for the Study of Intelligence. *Intelligence for a New Era in American Foreign Policy*. Washington, DC: Central Intelligence Agency, Center for the Study of Intelligence, January 2004.

Center for the Study of Intelligence. *Intelligence Lessons Learned Conference.* Washington, DC: Central Intelligence Agency, Center for the Study of Intelligence, May 2005.

Clift, A. Denis. "Intelligence in the Internet Era." *Studies in Intelligence* 47, no.3 (2003).

Congress of the United States, Public Law 108-458 (17 December 2004), "Intelligence Reform and Terrorism Prevention Act (IRTPA)."

Cooper, Jeffrey R. "Intelligence and Warning: Analytic Pathologies" (Powerpoint Briefing). SAIC, McLean, VA. November 2003.

———. "Sensemaking: Focusing on the Last Six Inches." Paper prepared for the American Institute of Aeronautics and Astronautics, Information and Command and Control Technical Committee, August 2002.

Cooper, Jeffrey R. and John Seely Brown. "Intelligence: We've Lost Our Edge." *Washington Post*, 10 May 2005.

Davis, Jack. *Improving CIA Analytic Performance: DI Analytic Priorities.* Sherman Kent Center for Intelligence Analysis, Occasional Papers, v.1, no. 3. Washington, DC: Central Intelligence Agency, September 2002.

———. *Improving CIA Analytic Performance: Strategic Warning.* Sherman Kent Center for Intelligence Analysis, Occasional Papers, v.1, no.1. Washington, DC: Central Intelligence Agency, September 2002.

———. "Paul Wolfowitz on Intelligence-Policy Relations," *Studies in Intelligence* 39, no. 1. (1995).

———. *Strategic Warning: If Surprise is Inevitable, What Role for Analysis?* Sherman Kent Center for Intelligence Analysis, Occasional Papers, v. 2, no.1. Washington, DC: Central Intelligence Agency, January 2003.

———. "The Kent-Kendall Debate of 1949." *Studies in Intelligence.* 35, no. 2 (1995).

Feschbach, Murray. *Russia's Health and Demographic Crises: Policy Implications and Consequences.* Chemical and Biological Arms Control Institute (Health and National Security Series), April 2003.

———. "Russia's Demographic and Health Meltdown." Congress of the United States, Joint Economic Committee, *Russia's Uncertain Economic Future,* 107th Congress, 1st Session. Washington, DC. Government Printing Office, December 2001.

Feinstein, Alvan R. *Clinical Judgment.* Baltimore, MD: Williams & Wilkins, 1967.

Fishbein, Warren, and Gregory Treverton. *Rethinking "Alternatives Analysis" to Address Transnational Threats.* Washington, DC: Central Intelligence Agency, The Sherman Kent Center for Intelligence Analysis, Occasional Papers, v. 3, no. 2, October 2004.

Goldhamer, Herbert. *The Adviser.* New York: Elsevier, 1978.

Goleman, Daniel, "Answer to 2005 Edge Question?" *The Edge.* http://edge.org/q2005/q05 print.html.

Hardin, Garrett. "The Tragedy of the Commons." *Science* 162 (1968): 1243–48.

Hayden, Michael V. (Lt. Gen., USAF). Statement Before the Joint Inquiry of the Senate Select Committee on Intelligence and the House Permanent Select Committee on Intelligence, 17 October 2002.

Heuer, Richards J., Jr. *The Psychology of Intelligence Analysis.* Washington, DC: Central Intelligence Agency, Center for the Study of Intelligence, 1999.

Hughes, Frank J., *Preparing for the Future of Intelligence Analysis.* Washington, DC: Joint Military Intelligence College, January 2003.

Hughes, Frank J. and David Schum. "Evidence Marshalling and Argument Construction." Washington, DC: Joint Military Intelligence College, Student Course Notes.

Jeremiah, David (Admiral, USN, ret.). Press Conference, CIA Headquarters, 2 June 1998.

———. *The Intelligence Community's Performance on the Indian Nuclear Tests* (1998).

Jervis, Robert. "What's Wrong with the Intelligence Process?" *International Journal of Intelligence and Counterintelligence* 1, no. 2 (Spring 1986).

Johnson, Loch. "The Aspin-Brown Intelligence Inquiry: Behind the Closed Doors of a Blue Ribbon Commission," *Studies in Intelligence* 48, no. 3 (2004).

Johnston, Rob. *Analytic Culture in the U.S. Intelligence Community: an Ethnographic Study.* Washington, DC: Central Intelligence Agency, Center for the Study of Intelligence, 2005

Kahneman, Daniel. Maps of Bounded Rationality: A Perspective on Intuitive Judgment and Choice. (Nobel) Prize Lecture, 8 December 2002. Princeton University, Department of Psychology.

———. Interview with author, October 2000.

Kahneman, Daniel, Paul Slovic, Amos Tversky, eds. *Judgment Under Uncertainty: Heuristics and Biases.* New York: Cambridge University Press, 1982.

Kent, Sherman, *Strategic Intelligence for American World Policy.* Princeton, NJ: Princeton University Press, 1951, revised edition 1966.

Kerbel, Josh. "Thinking Straight: Cognitive Bias in the US Debate on China," *Studies in Intelligence* 48, no. 3 (2004).

Kerr, Richard, Thomas Wolfe, Rebecca Donegan, and Aris Pappas. "Issues for the US Intelligence Community," *Studies in Intelligence* 49, no. 3 (2005).

———. Interview, MSNBC, 14 July 2003

Kissinger, Henry A. "America's Assignment," *Newsweek*, 8 November 2004.

———. "Better Intelligence Reform," *Washington Post*, 16 August 2004.

Klein, Gary. *Intuition at Work: Why Developing Your Gut Instinct Will Make You Better at What You Do.* New York: Doubleday, 2002.

Loomis, Carol. "Dinosaurs?" *Fortune*, 3 May 1993.

Marrin, Stephen. Review of William E. Odom, *Fixing Intelligence For a More Secure America, Political Science Quarterly* 119, no. 2 (Summer 2004).

———. "Preventing Intelligence Failures by Learning from the Past," *International Journal of Intelligence and Counterintelligence,* 17, No. 4 (Oct–Dec 2004).

MacEachin, Douglas. *CIA Assessments of the Soviet Union: The Record Versus the Charges.* Washington, DC: Central Intelligence Agency, Center for the Study of Intelligence, 1996.

McCarthy, Mary. "The National Warning System: Striving for an Elusive Goal," *Defense Intelligence Journal* 3, no. 1 (Spring 1994).

Mears, Michael. "The Intelligence Community Genome: RIA Paper #3." Unpublished manuscript, spring 2004.

Medawar, Peter. "Is the Scientific Paper Fraudulent? Yes; It Misrepresents Scientific Thought," *The Saturday Review*, 47, 1 August 1964.

Medina, Carmen. "What To Do When Traditional Models Fail," *Studies in Intelligence* 46, no. 3 (2002).

National Commission on Terrorist Attacks Upon the United States (The 9/11 Commission). *The 9/11 Commission Report: Final Report of the National Commission on Terrorist Attacks Upon the United States.* Washington, DC: Government Printing Office, 2004.

National Institute of Standards and Technology (NIST). *Dictionary of Algorithms and Data Structures.* http://www.nist.gov/dads.

Odom, William E. *Fixing Intelligence: for a More Secure America.* New Haven: Yale University Press, 2003.

Pappas, Aris A. and James M. Simon, Jr. "The Intelligence Community: 2001–2015," *Studies in Intelligence* 46, no.1 (2002).

Perrow, Charles. *Normal Accidents: Living with High-Risk Technologies.* New York: Basic Books, 1984.

Pfeffer, Jeffrey, with Charles A. O'Reilly. *Hidden Value: How Great Companies Achieve Extraordinary Results with Ordinary People.* Boston: Harvard Business School Press, 2000.

Pfeffer, Jeffrey, with G. R. Salancik. *The External Control of Organizations: A Resource Dependence Perspective.* New York: Harper and Row, 1978. (Republished by Stanford University Press, 2003.)

Principia Cybernetica Web. "Feedback." http://pespmc1.vub.ac.be/FEEDBACK.html (accessed 31 Aug 2005).

Rozak, David, Alexander Lee, James B. Petro, and Lisa Lechler. "Redefining the First Customer: Transforming Intelligence Analysis through Peer-Reviewed Publications" in 2004 Galileo Papers. Washington, DC: Central Intelligence Agency, 2005.

Rumsfeld, Donald. "Sideletter to Report of the Commission to Assess the Ballistic Missile Threat to the United States," 18 March 1991. http://www.house.gov/hasc/testimony/106thcongress/rumsfeldsideletter.htm.

S2845: An Act to Reform the Intelligence Community and the Intelligence and Intelligence-related Activities of the United States Government and for other purposes. (Short title: National Intelligence Reform Act of 2004.) 6 October 2004.

Sabel, Charles F. "Theory of a Real Time Revolution," forthcoming in *Organizational Studies* (2005). Forthcoming in Charles Heckscher, Paul Adler, eds., *Collaborative Community*. Oxford, UK: Oxford University Press, 2005.

Sageman, Mark. "Understanding Terror Networks," Foreign Policy Research Institute, E-Note, 1 November 2004. Available at http://www.fpri.org/enotes/20041101.middleeast. sageman.understandingterrornetworks.html.

Senate Select Committee on Intelligence of the 108th U.S. Congress. *Report on the US Intelligence Community's Prewar Intelligence Assessments.* Washington, DC: July 2004: 14. Available at: <http://www.realcities.com/multimedia/nationalchannel/news/ 070904_senate_report.pdf>.

Senge, Peter M. *The Fifth Discipline: The Art & Practice of the Learning Organization.* New York: Doubleday/Currency, 1990.

Shirky, Clay. "A Group Is Its Own Worst Enemy" (June 2003). "Networks, Economics, and Culture Mailing List." Available at http://www. shirky.com.

Simon, Herbert. *Administrative Behavior*. New York: The Free Press, 1997.
Six Sigma: <http://www.isixsigma.com/>

Stefik, Mark and Barbara Stefik. *Breakthrough: Stories and Strategies of Radical Innovation.* Cambridge, MA: MIT Press, 2004.

Stokes, Donald E. *Pasteur's Quadrant: Basic Science and Technology Innovation*. Washington, DC: The Brookings Institution, 1997.

Swenson, Russell and Susana C. Lemozy. "Politicization and Persuasion: Balancing Evolution and Devolution in Strategic Intelligence," unpublished manuscript (date?)

Travers, Russ. "The Coming Intelligence Failure," *Studies in Intelligence* 40, no. 2 (1996).

Warner, Michael. "Transformation and Intelligence Liaison," *SAIS Review of International Affairs* 24, no. 1 (Winter–Spring 2004).

Weick, Karl E. *Sensemaking in Organizations.* Thousand Oaks, CA: Sage Publications, 1995.

Weick, Karl E. and Kathleen M. Sutcliffe. *Managing the Unexpected: Assuring High Performance in an Age of Complexity.* San Francisco: Jossey-Bass, 2001.

INDEX

D

I

J

K

L

M

T

U

V

W

Y